Person-Centered Recovery Planner for Adults With Serious Mental Illness

Person-Centered Recovery Planner for Adults With Serious Mental Illness

Catherine N. Dulmus

Bruce C. Nisbet

WILEY

Cover Design: Andrew Liefer
Cover Image: © shaunl/iStockphoto

This book is printed on acid-free paper. ∞

Published by John Wiley & Sons, Inc., Hoboken, New Jersey.

Published simultaneously in Canada.

Limit of Liability/Disclaimer of Warranty: While the publisher and author have used their best efforts in preparing this book, they make no representations or warranties with respect to the accuracy or completeness of the contents of this book and specifically disclaim any implied warranties of merchantability or fitness for a particular purpose. No warranty may be created or extended by sales representatives or written sales materials. The advice and strategies contained herein may not be suitable for your situation. You should consult with a professional where appropriate. Neither the publisher nor author shall be liable for any loss of profit or any other commercial damages, including but not limited to special, incidental, consequential, or other damages.

This publication is designed to provide accurate and authoritative information in regard to the subject matter covered. It is sold with the understanding that the publisher is not engaged in rendering professional services. If legal, accounting, medical, psychological or any other expert assistance is required, the services of a competent professional person should be sought.

Designations used by companies to distinguish their products are often claimed as trademarks. In all instances where John Wiley & Sons, Inc. is aware of a claim, the product names appear in initial capital or all capital letters. Readers, however, should contact the appropriate companies for more complete information regarding trademarks and registration.

For general information on our other products and services please contact our Customer Care Department within the United States at (800) 762-2974, outside the United States at (317) 572-3993 or fax (317) 572-4002.

Wiley publishes in a variety of print and electronic formats and by print-on-demand. Some material included with standard print versions of this book may not be included in e-books or in print-on-demand. If this book refers to media such as a CD or DVD that is not included in the version you purchased, you may download this material at http://booksupport.wiley.com. For more information about Wiley products, visit www.wiley.com.

Library of Congress Cataloging-in-Publication Data

Dulmus, Catherine N.
  Person-centered recovery planner for adults with serious and persistent mental illness / Catherine N. Dulmus, Bruce C. Nisbet.
     pages cm
   Includes bibliographical references.
  ISBN 978-1-118-46435-9 (pbk. : acid-free paper)
  ISBN 978-1-118-65335-7 (ebk.)
  ISBN 978-1-118-65339-5 (ebk.)
  ISBN 978-1-118-65614-3 (ebk.)
  1. Mental illness--Treatment.–Planning–Handbooks, manuals, etc. 2. Chronic illness–Treatment–Planning–Handbooks, manuals, etc. 3. Psychotherapy–Planning–Handbooks, manuals, etc. I. Nisbet, Bruce C. II. Title.
  RC480.53.D85 2013
  616.89--dc23
                           2012049068

Printed in the United States of America
10 9 8 7 6 5 4 3 2 1

In loving memory of my daughter Abby
who always held tight to her
hopes and dreams.

—CND

Dedicated to my mother, grandmother, father, and
uncle who gave me the gift of a richly diverse
childhood in an extended-family home.

—BCN

CONTENTS

PREFACE

As friends and colleagues, we have had multiple conversations over the years about the challenges of preparing a workforce for a recovery-oriented practice, both from the perspectives of a social work educator and as a President/CEO of a community mental health agency. Our challenges were similar as we worked to prepare professionals to embrace person-centered planning within a recovery framework rather than the traditional top-down treatment planning approach when working with individuals with a serious mental illness. It was over dinner one evening that we once again had a conversation about recovery and the importance of moving the field forward, and it was where we came up with the idea of this recovery planner.

The field of mental health has become inundated with a variety of treatment planners, but they are not written as recovery planners incorporating person-centered planning and recovery-oriented principles that put the individual in charge of determining their own goals and their own path to recovery. With the publication of the *Person-Centered Recovery Planner for Adults with Serious Mental Illness*, practitioners now have a reference source to assist them in facilitating an individual developing their own person-centered recovery plan that meaningfully focuses on assisting them in achieving their hopes and dreams. This book will also be useful not only for the new practitioner but also the seasoned practitioner as they continue to build their creative approaches to being an effective person-centered facilitator and advocate for recovery. It will also serve well as both an undergraduate and graduate secondary textbook across disciplines (e.g., counseling, nursing, rehab, social work) that offer courses targeted to teaching students about working with individuals with serious mental illness.

Lastly, as Health Home care coordination programs are being established across the United States in response to incentives established under the Federal Affordable Care Act, the practices of person-centered recovery planning will need to be implemented as the most effective service approach to be used by these care coordination entities. The populations Health Homes exist to serve are high need Medicaid enrollees who are struggling with a serious mental illness and/or two or more chronic physical conditions. Enrollment by individuals is voluntary in these programs and person-centered recovery approaches will need to be utilized to build relationships that individuals will find engaging, empowering, and respectful. The *Person-Centered Recovery Planner for Adults with Serious Mental Illness* will be a valuable resource for these programs as they train their workforce in person-centered recovery planning in a Health Home care coordination environment.

We would like to extend our gratitude to the New York Care Coordination Project, Inc., who graciously allowed us to use many of their best practices and their Individual Service Plan forms within this book.

We also want to give a special thanks to Amy Millard, LCSW-R and Director of Intensive Services at Spectrum Human Services, Orchard Park, New York. Amy is a recognized expert in person-centered recovery planning and served as an invaluable consultant to us in the writing of this book. As she reviewed each draft chapter of this book her feedback consistently conveyed the profound respect and understanding of the recovery journeys of the multiple individuals she has worked with over the years. In the end Amy's valuable suggestions helped make this a better and more useful book for every reader.

Lastly we would like to thank our editor Marquita Flemming at John Wiley & Sons for her immediate enthusiasm for the recovery planner idea and for how quickly she moved the book proposal idea forward to contract.

We would be remiss not to acknowledge that our passion for persons with serious mental illness is a personal one, as we both have had family members who have been challenged by serious mental illness. We hope that this book will encourage and support practitioners in developing person-centered relationships with the persons they serve in order to embrace the hope and dreams of those they work with on their recovery journeys.

CATHERINE N. DULMUS
BRUCE C. NISBET

PART I
INTRODUCTION

CHAPTER 1   PERSON-CENTERED PRACTICE AND RECOVERY PRINCIPLES

Person-centered practice and recovery are relatively new orientations to working with people with serious mental illness; they have been transforming the field since their inception in the late 1980s and early 1990s. The 1970s championed deinstitutionalization that rightly resulted in people with serious mental illnesses being returned to their communities. Unfortunately, though, communities were often ill-prepared to welcome their neighbors home. More often than not, inadequate services and limited knowledge and understanding of mental illness abounded, which resulted in individuals being faced with significant stigma and little reason for hope.

The 1990s, however, brought person-centered practice and recovery principles, which continue to transform the field into one in which individuals receiving services have a voice and hope for recovery. These practices are empowering each person to define what recovery is for them and to be the decision makers in all aspects of their recovery planning and delivery of services. Organizations and their members who have been at the forefront of implementing recovery-oriented services include the New York Care Coordination Project, Inc., National Council for Community Behavioral Healthcare, and the Case Management Society of America.

WHAT IS PERSON-CENTERED PRACTICE?

Person-centeredness is about developing a relationship with another individual where the practitioner relates to that individual not as a diagnosis, not as someone who needs to be "fixed," but as another human being who desires to make changes in their life. It is a relationship in which the practitioner acts as a facilitator to assist that individual in moving forward on the changes and priorities that the *individuals* being served decide will improve their quality of life. As John O'Brien and Connie Lyle O'Brien (2002), leading thinkers on person-centered planning, have written, "Facilitation is a skillful process of realigning the energy around (the person)—eliciting, confirming, relating, summarizing, re-presenting, questioning, inviting, reflecting, focusing, pushing, encouraging, interpreting, checking out" (p. 16).

This book is written as a practical guide for new practitioners to support and encourage their own person-centered creativity as facilitators. More experienced practitioners will also find it useful as a desk reference when thinking about more complex sets of needs and desires on the part of individuals they are facilitating in the development and implementation of the individuals' recovery plan. The sample life goals, short-term objectives, and related recovery steps are only suggestions that are intended to prompt the practitioner's own creative thinking as a facilitator. Each recovery goal chapter suggests some life pathways and strategies that individuals being served can adapt to help themselves, when it fits their priorities. This is true whether they are at the beginning of their recovery journey, moving ahead, or at the point where they are ultimately leaving their practitioners behind as they progress on their own unique recovery paths and independence from ongoing paid mental health services and relationships. However, we also know that recovery is rarely a straight-line process, and it is always realistic to think that, even when individuals have reached a point where they have left their practitioners behind, periodically formal mental health services may be asked for or needed to assist individuals with their recovery journey.

When facilitating a recovery plan with individuals, it is the individuals who define what they deem to be their priority recovery goals. It is important to emphasize that the changes desired and priorities that are set are those of the individuals that are receiving services, and not those of the practitioner. Frankly, it is not important what the practitioner believes will improve the quality of life of individuals' they are working with but, rather, what the individuals see as the priorities to improve their own quality of life. Only in the case of health and safety or where individuals may be victims of abuse should practitioners take more direct and intervening roles to protect the individuals they are working with from harm. Otherwise, it is not the practitioners' place to decide; it is the responsibility of the individuals who are being helped to decide what their hopes and desires are. This includes the individuals' decisions about what objectives and recovery steps they choose to use in their recovery plan from those that have been offered or created within the working relationship. This is the essence of person-centered practice.

The New York State Care Coordination Program, Inc. (NYCCP), has been a regional and national leader in providing training and support for person-centered practice. Its website lists the following core values a practitioner must embrace to be person-centered in their practice (www.carecoordination.org/about_the_wnyccp.shtm):

- A commitment to know and to deeply seek to understand an individual.
- A conscious resolve to be of genuine service.
- Openness to being guided by the person.
- A willingness to struggle for difficult goals.
- A willingness to stand by values that enhance the humanity and dignity of the person.
- Flexibility, creativity, and openness to trying what might be possible, including innovation, experimentation, and unconventional solutions.
- To look for the good in people and help to bring it out.

The New York State Care Coordination Program, Inc., has also identified the hallmarks of person-centered practices that need to be evidenced by practitioners who are person-centered in their relationship and facilitation with individuals as follows (www.carecoordination.org/about_the_wnyccp.shtm):

- The person's activities, services, and supports are based upon his or her dreams, interest, preferences, and strengths.
- The person and people important to the person are included in lifestyle planning and have the opportunity to exercise control and make informed decisions.
- The person has meaningful choices, with decisions based on his or her experiences.
- The person uses, when possible, natural and community supports.
- Activities, supports, and services foster skills to achieve personal relationships, community inclusion, dignity, and respect.
- Planning is collaborative, recurring, and involves an ongoing commitment to the person.
- The person is satisfied with his or her activities, supports, and services.

The Person-Centered Recovery Planner for Adults with Serious Mental Illness is written to be consistent with these core values and hallmarks of person-centered practice. We seek to prompt and support the creative thinking and practice of a person-centered facilitator working with individuals in the development and implementation of their recovery plans.

WHAT IS RECOVERY?

There have been many definitions of mental health recovery for persons with serious mental illness since the findings of the President's New Freedom Commission on Mental Health in 2003. For the first time, the Commission embraced, at a national policy level, the concept that mental health recovery from serious mental illness was not only possible but, also, set as a priority that "care must focus on increasing consumers' ability to successfully cope with life's challenges, on facilitating recovery, and on building resilience" (President's New Freedom Commission on Mental Health, 2003, p. 2).

The current and probably the most widely embraced definition of recovery today, with the clearest articulation of the principles that support recovery, originates from the consensus results that the Substance Abuse and Mental Health Services Administration (SAMHSA) achieved at the federal level in 2010. In that year, SAMHSA brought together the broad cross-section of voices and perspectives discussed in more detail in the following section that achieved a very clear definition of recovery applicable to both mental health and substance use challenges. To that end we have included the results of those efforts here as we have written this recovery planner for practitioners to be consistent with the definition and principles of recovery detailed next. The overall intent of this recovery planner is to inform the reader of the opportunities, approaches, and challenges for practitioners that person-centered recovery planning offers and to prompt their creative thinking as facilitators in individuals' recovery journeys.

SAMHSA'S WORKING DEFINITION OF RECOVERY FOR MENTAL DISORDERS AND SUBSTANCE-USE DISORDERS

The Substance Abuse and Mental Health Services Administration (SAMHSA) recognizes there are many different pathways to recovery, and each individual determines his or her own way. SAMHSA engaged in a dialogue with consumers, persons in recovery, family members, advocates, policy makers, administrators, providers, and others to develop the following definition and guiding principles for recovery. The urgency of health reform compels SAMHSA to define recovery and to promote the availability, quality, and financing of vital services and supports that facilitate recovery for individuals. In addition, the integration mandate in title II of the Americans with Disabilities Act and the Supreme Court's decision in *Olmstead v. L.C.*, 527 U.S. 581 (1999) provide legal requirements that are consistent with SAMHSA's mission to promote a high-quality and satisfying life in the community for all Americans.

SAMHSA defines recovery from mental disorders and substance use disorders as a process of change through which individuals improve their health and wellness, live self-directed lives, and strive to reach their full potential. Through the Recovery Support Strategic Initiative, SAMHSA has delineated four major dimensions that support life in recovery as:

1. *Health:* overcoming or managing one's disease(s) as well as living in a physically and emotionally healthy way.
2. *Home:* a stable and safe place to live.
3. *Purpose:* meaningful daily activities, such as a job, school, volunteerism, family caretaking, or creative endeavors, and the independence, income, and resources to participate in society.
4. *Community:* relationships and social networks that provide support, friendship, love, and hope. (SAMHSA, 2011)

SAMSHA'S GUIDING PRINCIPLES OF RECOVERY

Recovery emerges from hope: The belief that recovery is real provides the essential and motivating message of a better future, that people can and do overcome the internal and external challenges, barriers, and obstacles that confront them. Hope is internalized and can be fostered by peers, families, providers, allies, and others. Hope is the catalyst of the recovery process.

Recovery is person driven: Self-determination and self-direction are the foundations for recovery as individuals define their own life goals and design their unique path(s) toward those goals. Individuals optimize their autonomy and independence to the greatest extent possible by leading, controlling, and exercising choice over the services and supports that assist their recovery and resilience. In so doing, they are empowered and provided the resources to make informed decisions, initiate recovery, build on their strengths, and gain or regain control over their lives.

Recovery occurs via many pathways: Individuals are unique with distinct needs, strengths, preferences, goals, culture, and backgrounds, including trauma experiences, that affect and determine their pathway(s) to recovery. Recovery is built on the multiple capacities, strengths, talents, coping abilities, resources, and inherent value of each individual. Recovery pathways are highly personalized. They may include professional clinical treatment; use of medications; support from families and in schools; faith-based approaches; peer support; and other approaches. Recovery is nonlinear, characterized by continual growth and improved functioning that may involve setbacks. Because setbacks are a natural, though not inevitable, part of the recovery process, it is essential to foster resilience for all individuals and families. Abstinence is the safest approach for those with substance use disorders. Use of tobacco and nonprescribed or illicit drugs is not safe for anyone. In some cases, recovery pathways can be enabled by creating a supportive environment. This is especially true for children, who may not have the legal or developmental capacity to set their own course.

Recovery is holistic: Recovery encompasses an individual's whole life, including mind, body, spirit, and community. This includes addressing: self-care practices, family, housing, employment, education, clinical treatment for mental disorders and substance use disorders, services and supports, primary health care, dental care, complementary and alternative services, faith, spirituality, creativity, social networks, transportation, and community participation. The array of services and supports available should be integrated and coordinated.

Recovery is supported by peers and allies: Mutual support and mutual aid groups, including the sharing of experiential knowledge and skills, as well as social learning, play an invaluable role in recovery. Peers encourage and engage other peers and provide each other with a vital sense of belonging, supportive relationships, valued roles, and community. By helping others and giving back to the community, people help themselves. Peer-operated supports and services provide important resources to assist people along their journeys of recovery and wellness. Professionals can also play an important role in the recovery process by providing clinical treatment and other services that support individuals in their chosen recovery paths. Although peers and allies play an important role for many in recovery, their role for children and youth may be slightly different. Peer supports for families are very important for children with behavioral health problems and can also play a supportive role for youth in recovery.

Recovery is supported through relationship and social networks: An important factor in the recovery process is the presence and involvement of people who believe in the person's ability to recover; who offer hope, support, and encouragement; and who also suggest strategies and resources for change. Family members, peers, providers, faith groups, community members, and other allies form vital support networks. Through these relationships, people leave unhealthy and/or unfulfilling life roles behind and engage in new roles (e.g., partner, caregiver, friend, student, employee) that lead to a greater sense of belonging, personhood, empowerment, autonomy, social inclusion, and community participation.

Recovery is culturally based and influenced: Culture and cultural background in all its diverse representations, including values, traditions, and beliefs, are keys in determining a person's journey and unique pathway to recovery. Services should be culturally grounded, attuned, sensitive, congruent, and competent, as well as personalized to meet each individual's unique needs.

Recovery is supported by addressing trauma: The experience of trauma (such as physical or sexual abuse, domestic violence, war, disaster, and others) is often a precursor to or associated with alcohol and drug use, mental health problems, and related issues. Services and supports should be trauma informed to foster safety (physical and emotional) and trust, as well as to promote choice, empowerment, and collaboration.

Recovery involves individual, family, and community strengths and responsibility: Individuals, families, and communities have strengths and resources that serve as a foundation for recovery. In addition, individuals have personal responsibilities for their own self-care and journeys of recovery. Individuals should be supported in speaking for themselves. Families and significant others have responsibilities to support their loved ones, especially for children and youth in recovery. Communities have responsibilities to provide opportunities and resources to address discrimination and to foster social inclusion and recovery. Individuals in recovery also have a social responsibility and should have the ability to join with peers to speak collectively about their strengths, needs, wants, desires, and aspirations.

Recovery is based on respect: Community, systems, and societal acceptance and appreciation for people affected by mental health and substance use problems, including protecting their rights and eliminating discrimination, are crucial in achieving recovery. There is a need to acknowledge that taking steps toward recovery may require great courage. Self-acceptance, developing a positive and meaningful sense of identity, and regaining belief in oneself are particularly important.

SAMHSA has developed this working definition of recovery to help policy makers, providers, funders, peers/consumers, and others design, measure, and reimburse for integrated and holistic services and supports to more effectively meet the individualized needs of those served. Many advances have been made to promote recovery concepts and practices. There are a variety of effective models and practices that states, communities, providers, and others can use to promote recovery. However, much work remains to ensure that recovery-oriented behavioral-health services and systems are adopted and implemented in every state and community. Drawing on research, practice, and personal experience of recovering individuals, within the context of health reform, SAMHSA will lead efforts to advance the understanding of recovery and ensure that vital recovery supports and services are available and accessible to all who need and want them (SAMHSA, 2011).

PERSON-CENTERED PRACTICE AND RECOVERY

As this chapter indicates, the principles of person-centered practice and recovery complement each other and together provide a powerful framework for working with individuals with serious mental illness. This approach to practice supports individuals as unique persons and empowers them to define what recovery means for them and the priorities and steps to moving forward.

REFERENCES

New York State Care Coordination Program, Inc. (n.d.). Retrieved September 14, 2013 from http://www.carecoordination.org/about-nyccp.aspx

O'Brien, J., & O'Brien, C. (2002). *Implementing person-centered planning: Voices of experience.* Toronto, Canada: Inclusion Press.

President's New Freedom Commission on Mental Health. (2003). *Achieving the promise: Transforming mental health care in America.* DHHS Pub. No. SMA-03-3831. Rockville, MD.

SAMSHA. (2011). Retrieved from http://blog.samhsa.gov/2011/12/22/samhsa%E2%80%99s-definition-and-guiding-principles-of-recovery-%E2%80%93-answering-the-call-for-feedback/

CHAPTER 2 PERSON-CENTERED ASSESSMENT AND INDIVIDUAL SERVICE PLANNING FOR RECOVERY

PERSON-CENTERED ASSESSMENT

Assessment is typically the first opportunity for a practitioner to begin to build a person-centered relationship with individuals referred for services. Individuals should be encouraged to bring to this first meeting any family, friends, peers, providers, or others whom they wish to have involved in their recovery assessment/planning. A confidentiality release needs to be signed by the individual naming anyone they wish to include in their planning.

Assessment occurs as a conversation that epitomizes the very first core value of person-centered practice as cited in Chapter 1: "A commitment to know and to deeply seek to understand an individual." A person-centered assessment conversation begins with exploring and understanding the individual's strengths, skills, talents, capacities, areas of health, and protective factors that have contributed to that person's past and present successes in achieving some of his or her life goals. These strengths and successes will continue to be critical resources for the individual to draw on to support the achievement of identified current life goal priorities and preferences on the individual's continuing recovery journey.

The assessment conversation needs to go on to explore barriers to achieving recovery goals. Potential barriers might be due to formal system limitations or rigidity, the individual's physical and behavioral health needs, or treatment experiences and preferences past and present. In addition, the assessment conversation needs to explore social and environmental needs (such as housing) and preferences, natural (family, friends, neighbors), informal (nonpaid resources), and formal (paid resources) supports that are or are not currently in place, and overall should be comprehensive enough to clearly define what the individual's preferences are, and what identified needs and desires are for services and initial goals. A well-done person-centered assessment creates the basis for beginning to build trust and a partnership to develop an initial Individualized Service Plan (ISP), sometimes also referred to as an Individualized Action Plan (IAP), that communicates to the individual that his or her desires and preferences are valued and will lead the process. Because the path to recovery and life in general can create stresses and challenges for some individuals that can lead to a mental health crisis needing temporary support, the development of a well-thought out Crisis Plan in advance by the individual being served should always be a part of the ISP planning process.

USING THE RECOVERY PLANNER

Following the completion of the person-centered assessment in which the individual has determined what his or her priority life goals are to focus on, the next task for practitioners is to partner with the individual in facilitating the development, in the individual's own words, his or her ISP. By design, the ISP is the individual's own unique path to continuing recovery.

It is here that the recovery planner is a resource for practitioners to prompt their creative thinking in their role as person-centered facilitators and advocates. It provides a range of objectives and recovery steps for practitioners to offer individuals to choose from in each of their life goal areas that are the individuals' priority. Each recovery goal chapter also has blank lines throughout for practitioners to further customize their approaches. Practitioners need to tailor the recovery steps they offer individuals to be consistent with the existing capacity, knowledge, strengths, and skills that individuals already brings to the process. Some individuals are at the *beginning* stage of exploring and learning what they can choose from in terms of available or created informal and/or formal supports, and engaging in developing the skills and confidence needed to make use of them. Some individuals may already be at the *moving forward* stage and may need some additional support to fully engage in their identified informal and formal resources or, when the individual is not satisfied with their informal and/or formal supports currently in place, ask practitioners to facilitate alternative options. Finally, some individuals will already be at the beginning stage of *leaving their practitioners behind* and need to further build their confidence that their independence from practitioners' services is right for them.

In using the Recovery Planner, the practitioner needs to assess with the individual where the individual is in their pursuit of each of their identified priority life goals and tailor their suggested objectives and recovery steps to the individual's preferences and needs. The practitioner also needs to listen closely to the individual as to what are their own suggestions for objectives and recovery steps and incorporate those into the plan. In the end it is the individual's ISP and they get to choose what they assess is the right "fit" for them and benefit from the results and learning that occurs as they implement their ISP for recovery. In this way completing the ISP is a mutually creative process where the practitioner and the individual can partner together. The *Person-Centered Recovery Planner for Adults with Serious Mental Illness* is intended as a support for the creativity and experience both the practitioner and individual bring to the development of the individual's ISP and overall recovery plan. It is also written in a manner designed to remind the practitioner they are a facilitator, a navigator, a guide . . . not a decider. The person they are working with is in charge of choosing what *they* determine will be the most helpful to them in their recovery journey.

Last but not least, each practitioner must remember that as person-centered facilitators they need to evidence, in their practice, the core values of person-centeredness as outlined in Chapter 1. These include flexibility, creativity, and openness to trying what might be possible, including innovation, experimentation, and nontraditional solutions. This recovery planner is a starting point but it is not a substitute for practitioners' own flexibility, creativity, and openness in the planning process. It is also imperative that practitioners embrace their responsibility to be advocates for formal systems to adapt to meet the individuals' needs, rather than expecting the individual to fit into existing services, programs, or structures based on erroneous assumptions that individuals must have certain "generic needs" that can be addressed by a one-size-fits-all mentality. Practitioners must also realize that the service system is limited, and that they must often creatively reach outside the service system to be an effective facilitator.

DEVELOPING A PERSON-CENTERED RECOVERY PLAN

Introduction

All organizations that engage in person-centered recovery planning will have developed their version of an Individual Service Plan (ISP) for recovery and may even call it by a different name. For the purposes of this book, the ISP for recovery format contained later in this chapter is utilized by Spectrum Human Services, Orchard Park, New York, in their Care Coordination Program. This program provides person-centered recovery services for individuals referred who have a serious mental illness that is: interfering with their reaching one or more of their life goals, impacting their quality of life and interfering with their ability to maintain themselves in the community. Spectrum has been a leader in the provision of person-centered recovery planning with thousands of individuals during the course of its 20 years as a care-coordination provider, and has had a high level of success with facilitating individuals in their recovery journeys.

This ISP format was developed collaboratively among several care-coordination agencies in Erie County, New York, including Spectrum, and it was adopted by the New York Care Coordination Project, Inc., for use in several other western New York counties. At any one time, approximately 3,000 individuals are utilizing this ISP across the western portion of the state. The ISP forms are available at no cost for download at http://www.carecoordination.org/care_coordination_forms.shtm. This is the website of the New York Care Coordination Project, Inc., whose mission includes the dissemination of best practices in person-centered recovery planning.

CREATING A PERSON-CENTERED ISP FOR RECOVERY

In this section of the chapter, we provide an example of how to create a person-centered ISP for recovery. A case study is provided and then applied to the ISP process and forms that are available at the end of the book as well as at the website previously mentioned. In doing this example, we provide one recovery goal as an illustration of how to use the ISP with this recovery planner.

John Smith Referral Summary

John Smith is a 49-year-old individual who was referred for care-coordination services. His referral states that he has just been discharged from in-patient psychiatric services following a recent suicide attempt and running from the police. He is linked by the hospital with an outpatient therapist, but he has a history of frequent hospitalizations due to suicide attempts and a lack of follow-through with his outpatient appointments. He is frequently homeless due to losing his monthly SSI money through gambling and subsequently not paying his rent. John has a brother who has been very involved in providing needed support for him. John's referral states that his Axis I diagnosis is Major Depressive Disorder, Severe, Recurrent with many unresolved trauma issues regarding the murder of his son 6 years ago.

Step One

The practitioner is able to reach John and arranges to meet him at his apartment. The role of care coordination, the assessment process, and the ISP process are described to him. John agrees to participate and is encouraged to have any family, friends, peers, or others (natural supports) he might choose join him to attend the next meeting and be part of the person-centered assessment process. John identifies his brother as someone he wants to be involved, and the assessment meeting is set to occur at John's apartment.

Step Two

At the beginning of the meeting at John's apartment, he signs a release for his brother to be involved and the practitioner completes the person-centered assessment as a conversation described in the beginning of this chapter. The practitioner also completes a risk assessment with John and determines John's current risk for self-harm is at a moderate level. (Risk assessments are recommended to be done at least every 6 months as well at any point that there are significant life events and/or stressors that could impact an individual's lethality level.) Releases are also signed by John to get his records from the hospital and former therapists/medical doctors. John's brother has and will be an important support and resource for him. John has identified six goals that he wants to pursue in his recovery journey through his ISP.

At the end of the assessment conversation, the practitioner reviews with John the introductory page of the ISP, which explains how the service planning works. This introduction reinforces that the planning is person-centered by virtue of examples of how John will he leading the choices and development of the plan. John completes (in his own words and with the help of the practitioner, if needed) Part A – Participant's Personal Profile of the ISP. The practitioner documents the completion of

Part A and any subsequent updates of Part A (practitioner reviews with the individual and updates as necessary at least every 6 months) are documented on that portion of the form labeled "Update Information," which immediately follows the last section of the Part A form labeled "Discharge Criteria." John agrees that initially he would prioritize three of his goals to work on because he expressed concerns about being overwhelmed by more than three at a time (in our experience this is the recommended maximum number of goals for individuals to work on concurrently). A next meeting is set at his brother's house to address developing his initial ISP together.

Step Three

The practitioner writes his/her assessment back at the office, based on the assessment conversation with John and his brother. Knowing John's first three preferred goals, the practitioner uses the recovery planner to prompt his/her own thinking and creative ideas about objectives and associated recovery steps that could be offered to John in each of his goal areas. Those ideas are written down by practitioner in his/her notes to refer to during the upcoming ISP development meeting.

Step Four

The practitioner meets with John at his brother's house. John is very engaged and the practitioner facilitates John completing (in his own words) his first three priority goals, objectives, and preferred recovery steps. John's first goal, objective, and recovery steps are illustrated in the sample ISP form labeled "Part B–Participant's Recovery Goal, Objective, and Recovery Steps." Work done by both John and the practitioner, respectively, to implement the recovery steps are documented by both under "Ongoing Updates" on the Part B form.

Step Five

The final step in the ISP process is for John to complete "Part C – Participant's Crisis Prevention Plan" as illustrated in the sample form. Each crisis-prevention plan should be reviewed regularly (at least every 6 months or at sentinel events) with the individual, and updates documented as shown as the crisis-prevention plan is developed, reviewed, and updated.

Step Six

In conclusion, the ISP should be considered by both the practitioner and the individual being served as a living, dynamic vehicle for facilitating an individual's recovery journey. As such, the ISP needs ongoing modification in response to both an individual's successes as well as the individual's challenges in achieving his or her recovery goals.

INDIVIDUAL SERVICE PLAN FOR RECOVERY

You and your Care Coordinator have the opportunity to work together on an Individual Service Plan (ISP) and a Crisis Prevention Plan. You may also want a friend, a family member, and/or a valued provider included in the development of this plan.

Services in the plan may include mental health and/or chemical dependency treatment, housing and financial assistance, and any other things that you identify as a support. You can also address life areas that you are not satisfied with or need more help with. You may want to set goals and develop a service plan that addresses some or all of the following life areas:

Recovery & Rehabilitation   **Self-Help & Empowerment**

Physical Health & Wellness   **Educational & Employment**

Financial   **Legal**

Housing   **Spirituality**

Community Presence & Participation   **Other** _____

You may write a plan with as many goals and services as you want. You may review the plan and add goals and services at any time by talking about this with your Care Coordinator.

As you work with your Care Coordinator on the Individual Service Plan, you will want to consider what personal supports and community resources can help you achieve your goals, what services and which service providers have been most helpful in the past, what prevents you from getting and keeping what you need, and what strengths, supports and experiences you can use to achieve your goals. Your Care Coordinator will assist you in accessing the services, supports, and organizations that you need in order to carry out your plan.

Your Care Coordinator will also work with you to develop a Crisis Prevention Plan. This plan will help you recognize situations and people that may cause you stress, and identify people and things that may help you to relieve stress.

Part A – Participant's Personal Profile
(As established in the Assessment)

Values and areas of interest (Things that are important to me: hopes, dreams, interests)

"God is important to me. I like to work out. My nieces are important to me. I want to feel happy instead of miserable. I want better transportation to get to my counselor and around. I want to learn to eat better. I want to stop gambling my money away. I want to not be in pain with my leg. I want a job."

Strengths (Skills, qualities, and experiences that can help me achieve my goals)

"I am a good worker. I like to work out and take care of myself. I can make people laugh "

Personal and community supports (People and/or things I have in my life that can help me achieve my goals)

"My brother. My pastor."

Possible barriers (Things that could prevent me from achieving these goals)

"My gambling, hurting myself, no money for buses, no doctor, didn't get my high school diploma"

Discharge criteria (How I will know that I don't need Care Coordination anymore)

"When I feel like I am ready to be on my own"

Date	Update Information	Participant Initials	Provider Initials
10/06/2012	Met with John at his apartment & completed his Initial Assessment with him. He filled out his Personal Profile after our conversation and we discussed doing his Individual Service Plan at our next meeting. He wants his brother involved in his planning. John has identified six priority life goals. Will meet in 2 weeks to do ISP.	JS (signed)	BCN (signed)
	NOTE: Utilize this form for documenting that the initial Personal Profile was completed by the person served in their own words based on their initial assessment conversation. Reassessment updates of the Personal Profile with the individual (every 3 or 6 months) are documented on this form and utilizing for space the next "Part A Continued" form.		

Participant Name: John Smith   Care Coordination Program: Spectrum Human Services
ID: 345678   DOB: 5/23/1963   Date of Plan: 10/06/2012

Part A – Participant's Personal Profile (continued)
(As established in the Assessment)

Date	Update Information	Participant Initials	Provider Initials
	(See Note on prior page)		

Copy this page as often as needed to provide updates to the participant's personal profile.

Reproduced by Permission of the New York Care Coordination Project, Inc.

Participant Name: John Smith
ID: 345678   DOB: 5/23/1963   Date of Plan: 10/06/2012

Part B – Participant's Recovery Goal, Objective, and Recovery Steps

Goal #1 Participant's Recovery Goal Expressed in Their Own Words: "I want to have better transportation"

Development Date: 10/20/12

Barriers (What is getting in the way of achieving the goal as per assessment)

"Spending my money on cards, pool"

"Giving my money away. I don't budget well"

Strengths (Existing supports for achieving the goal)

"I know how to get around on buses. I was receiving a bus pass before from somewhere but I am not sure where"

Objective # 1 (Step toward the goal and how I will know I have accomplished this)

"I want to get a bus pass"

Effective Date: 10/20/12   Target Completion Date: 11/5/12

RECOVERY STEPS - Specific Services/Activities/Supports/Tasks (What I and/or others will do to achieve this objective)	Who is Responsible (Person/s who will provide the service or carry out the task)	Start Date	Target Completion Date	Frequency (How often to meet)	Service $ Expense (CK if yes)
Care Coordinator (CC) will provide services by providing options for John to choose from to receive a bus pass	Care Coordinator	10/20/2012	10/20/2012	Meet at least 2X monthly	No
CC will provide linkage to the public bus company reduced fare card program per John's choice	Care Coordinator	10/20/2012	11/5/2012	1X	No
CC will provide linkage for John for budgeting classes and/or a representative payee to temporarily assist his managing his money based on his choice. Care Coordinator will monitor the plan for follow-through and satisfaction	Care Coordinator	10/20/2012	12/1/2012	2X/month	No
CC will assess for any barriers and plan to assist John removing any barriers if he requests assistance	Care Coordinator	10/20/2012	12/1/2012	2X/month	No
I will try to budget my money better; I will apply for a reduced bus pass; I will purchase a bus pass at the beginning of each month on the day I get my check; I will decide if I want a rep payee or not	Self	10/20/2012	12/1/2012	Meet at least 2X monthly	No

Ongoing Updates

Date	Progress	Achievement Code C (continue) A-Achieved D-Discontinue R-Revised	Participant Initials	Provider Initials
11/5/2012	Reviewed reduced fare application with John and he completed today. Objective will continue until approval is received and John has picture card to use. Target date 12/1/2012.	C	JS (signed)	BCN (signed)
11/19/2012	Objective reviewed today and will continue as John has not received his approval letter or had his picture taken. This objective will continue. New target date is 1/5/2013. He wants to go to budgeting class when he gets his bus pass. CC will link him then.		JS (signed)	BCN (signed)

Copy this page as often as needed to create new goals and/or objectives. Attach additional pages (see next page) as needed to provide updates to this goal and/or objective.

Reproduced by Permission of the New York Care Coordination Project, Inc.

Part B – Participant's Recovery Goal, Objective, and Recovery Steps (continued)

Goal # 1   Participant's Recovery Goal, Objective, and Recovery Steps (continued)
and around"

**Goal # 1   Participant's Desired Outcome: "I want to have better transportation to get to my counselor
and around"**

Development Date: 10/20/2012   Objective # 1 (Step toward the goal and how I will know I have accomplished this) **"I want to
get a bus pass"**

Effective Date: 10/20/12   Target Completion Date: 11/5/12

12/3/2012	Objective reviewed today and will continue as John has not received his approval letter yet or had his picture taken. This objective will continue until he receives his ID card for reduced fare bus transportation. Target date remains 1/5/2013.	C	JS (signed) BCN (signed)
12/17/2012	John has received his approval letter and plans to get his picture taken on 12/22/2012. New target date is 1/20/2013.	C	JS (signed) BCN (signed)
1/5/2013	John got his picture taken and sent it in to the bus company. He is waiting for his Medicaid reduced fare bus pass. Target date remains 1/20/2013.	C	JS (signed) BCN (signed)

Participant Name: John Smith
ID: 345678   DOB: 5/23/1963   Date of Plan: 10/06/2012

Care Coordination Program: Spectrum Human Services

		A	JS (signed)	BCN (signed)
1/10/2013	John received his reduced fare bus pass last week and is using it daily. Objective achieved.			

Copy this page as often as needed to provide updates to this goal and/or objective.

Reproduced by Permission of the New York Care Coordination Project, Inc.

Participant Name: John Smith
ID: 345678   DOB: 5/23/1963   Date of Plan: 10/06/2012

Care Coordination Program: Spectrum Human Services

PART C – PARTICIPANT'S CRISIS PREVENTION PLAN

If the participant has a Wellness Recovery Action Plan™ (WRAP), it may be attached and this form used only for additional or updated information.

HEALTH CARE PROXY HAS BEEN EXECUTED? (x) Yes ( ) No	OTHER ADVANCE DIRECTIVE HAS BEEN EXECUTED? ( ) Yes (x) No	WELLNESS RECOVERY ACTION PLAN™ (WRAP) HAS BEEN EXECUTED? ( ) Yes (x) No
(x) Copy Attached	Copy Attached	Copy Attached
Document Location: **Spectrum file** **Brother** Does the Participant have a copy? (x) Yes ( ) No	If No: ___ Need More Information ___ Refused (state reason below)	Document Location: Does the Participant have a copy? ( ) Yes ( ) No	If No: ___ Need More Information **X** Refused (state reason below) **States does not need it**	Document Location: Does the Participant have a copy? ( ) Yes ( ) No	If No: ___ Need More Information **X** Refused (state reason below) **States does not need it**

MY CRISIS PREVENTION PLAN: (How can I avoid a crisis?):

Take my Meds   Exercising
Going to treatment

Are there people, places, or things I should avoid? What are they?
Pool halls, casinos, card games

What are my early warning signs?
Talking suicidal   Not being able to sleep
Wanting to give up

My CRISIS PLAN (What can be done if I am in crisis?)

Call for help

Ways I can relieve stress, regain balance, calm myself, or make myself safer:

Work out, watch TV, volunteer, be with or call friends or those who care, play with my cat

Persons I can call:
My brother – 555-1212
My Pastor – 555-1212

Resources I can use:
Spectrum Care Coordinator (555-1212)   My counselor (555-1212)
Crisis Services hot line (555-1212)   Peer "warm" line to talk (555-1212)

Things I or others can do that I find helpful or keep me safe:

Meet with me more often, see my counselor more often, avoid upsetting things, volunteering, taking walks.

Medications that have helped in the past:	Medications that have not helped:	Types of medication(s) I take:
Wellbutrin	Not sure	Wellbutrin

Participant Name: John Smith
Care Coordination Program: Spectrum Human Services

ID: 345678   DOB: 5/23/1963   Date of Plan: 10/06/2012

PART C – PARTICIPANT'S CRISIS PREVENTION PLAN (CONTINUED)

IF I BECOME UNABLE TO HANDLE MY PERSONAL AFFAIRS, the following people have agreed to look after my personal affairs
(For example: pets, housing, family/job notification):

Name	Phone	Area(s) of Assistance
Peter Smith (Brother)	716-555-1212	Check on my apartment so things are okay. Feed my cat named Morris. Tell my doctors what I want and don't want. Take care of my money and pay rent and bills. Health Care Proxy
Pastor Edward Kryder	716-555-1212	Come see me so he can talk to me and pray for me.

I have developed this Crisis Plan to describe the actions that I would like to take place should I be in a crisis situation.

Participant's Signature: John Smith (signed)   **Date:** 10/20/2012

Ongoing Updates

Review Date	Update/Comment	Participant Initials	Provider Initials
10/20/2012	John developed his first Crisis Plan. We will review regularly.	JS (signed)	BCN (signed)
	Attach additional pages (see next page) as needed to provide updates to the Crisis Prevention Plan.		

Reproduced by Permission of the New York Care Coordination Project, Inc.

PART C – PARTICIPANT'S CRISIS PREVENTION PLAN (CONTINUED)

Ongoing Updates

Review Date	Update / Comment	Participant Initials	Provider Initials
	(Note: Use this form for continuing documentation of ongoing updates/reviews with John on his Crisis Plan)		

Copy this page as often as needed to provide updates to the Crisis Prevention Plan.

Participant Name: John Smith
ID: 345678   DOB: 5/23/1963   Date of Plan: 10/06/2012

ASSESSMENT/PLAN SUMMARY/REVIEW – SIGNATURE PAGE

TYPE: Initial Plan: **X**   Periodic Review 3 mo. _____   Periodic Review 6 mo. _____   Other Review _____   Date: 10/6/2012

Participant Comments (Comment on progress toward goals and topics that require further discussion and/or services that might be further explored.)

I am happy with my plan. I think it will help me.

Provider Comments (Provide a brief summary of the plan, including identified areas of concern that are not in the ISP, reasons for not including them at this time, and what, if any future actions will be taken to include them. Use this summary to update the assessment, as required.)

John has identified six priority life areas/goals that he wants to pursue. He has chosen to work on his three highest need goals ("I want to feel happy instead of miserable; I want better transportation to get to my counselor and around; I want to stop gambling my money away") first and add the others as he accomplishes the first three so he would not be overwhelmed.

Signatures of Individuals Contributing to the Individual Service Plan: Copies of Plan Provided To:

Signatures of Individuals Contributing to the Individual Service Plan	Copies of Plan Provided To
Participant Signature: JS (signed)	Participant Name: John Smith
Date: 10/6/2012	Date: 10/6/2012
Care Coordinator Signature: BCN (signed)	Care Coordinator Name: BCN
Date: 10/06/2012	Date: 10/6/2012
Service Provider Signature: TN (signed – therapist with JS written release)	Service Provider Name: TN(with JS written release)
Date: 10/12/2012	Date: 10/12/2012
Other Signature (specify): Peter Smith (brother)	Other Name (specify): Peter Smith
Date: 10/06/2012	Date: 10/06/2012

Reproduced by Permission of the New York Care Coordination Project, Inc.

PART II
RECOVERY GOALS

CHAPTER 3   MENTAL HEALTH AND CO-OCCURRING SUBSTANCE ABUSE SUPPORTS

A mental health and co-occurring substance abuse supports goal is developed by individuals to assist them with identifying and obtaining the most effective mental health and, as applicable, substance abuse supports available. Where mental health and substance abuse are co-occurring, integrated treatment creates the best opportunity to achieve optimal mental health in support of recovery.

INDIVIDUAL'S RECOVERY FOCUS

1. Good mental health as defined by the individual in his or her own words.

___. _____

   _____

___. _____

   _____

BEGINNINGS

Individual's current status

1. No mental health or co-occurring supports in place.
2. Minimal mental health or co-occurring supports in place.
3. Adequate mental health or co-occurring supports in place.
4. Dissatisfied with current mental health or co-occurring supports.

___. _____

   _____

___. _____

   _____

Short-term objectives

1. Individual identifies if they have any current mental health or substance abuse symptoms that are negatively impacting his or her quality of life.
2. Individual expresses in his or her own words his or her hopes and dreams for mental health, including substance use.
3. Individual provides history of informal and formal mental health and substance abuse supports utilized.
4. Individual identifies what (if any) current informal and formal mental health and, as applicable, substance abuse supports are in place and satisfaction with supports.
5. Individual identifies whether his or her current mental health and substance abuse treatment is integrated with the same treatment provider.
6. Individual identifies any prescribed medications by a mental health provider and, if so, the individual's current engagement and satisfaction with medication regime.
7. Individual identifies his or her strengths and specific capacities to achieving good mental health.
8. Individual identifies any obstacles and/or barriers that are negatively impacting his or her engagement with current mental health and, as applicable, substance abuse supports.
9. Individual identifies any natural supports (family/significant others and/or friends) that would like to be involved in the development of his or her mental health and, as applicable, substance abuse support recovery goal.
10. Individual expresses his or her mental health support goal including substance use, as applicable, in his or her own words.
11. Individual chooses to move forward on his or her mental health supports recovery goal.

____. _____

_____

____. _____

_____

____. _____

_____

Recovery steps

1. Individual identifies any current symptoms that are negatively impacting their quality of life.
2. Educate individual on all available crisis services in the community.
3. Explore with individual their hopes and dreams regarding their mental health and, as applicable, substance use.
4. Support individual in expressing his or her mental health and, as applicable, co-occurring substance abuse supports goal in his or her own words.
5. Individual lists detailed history of informal and formal mental health and, as applicable, substance abuse supports they have utilized.
6. Determine with individual their veteran status and any use of veterans' programs.
7. Obtain list of all current mental health and, as applicable, substance abuse supports in place.
8. Determine with individual his or her satisfaction with each current mental health and, as applicable, substance abuse supports.
9. Individual identifies the frequency and intensity of his or her participation in each of their current mental health/substance abuse supports.
10. Assist individual in identifying and listing his or her strengths and capacities that support achieving good mental health.
11. Identify any barriers that are impeding individual's engagement with one or more of his or her current mental health/substance abuse supports.
12. Identify with individual any natural supports he or she would like included in development of their mental health/co-occurring substance abuse supports recovery goal.
13. With written permission, include identified natural supports in recovery-goal planning meetings as individual desires.
14. Identify with individual mental health peer support and, if applicable, co-occurring mutual self-help programs in community.
15. Individual chooses to move forward on his or her mental health and co-occurring supports recovery goal.

___. _____
    _____
___. _____
    _____

_____. _____
        _____
_____. _____
        _____
_____. _____
        _____

MOVING FORWARD

Individual's current status

1. Individual is not in crisis.
2. Individual has expressed his or her mental health and co-occurring substance abuse supports recovery goal in his or her own words.
3. Individual has identified any current mental health/substance abuse symptoms that are negatively impacting his or her quality of life.
4. Individual has provided mental health and, as applicable, substance abuse supports history.
5. Veteran information determined.
6. Current mental health and, if applicable, substance abuse supports identified.
7. Individual's engagement and satisfaction with current medication regime determined.
8. Individual's satisfaction and level of engagement with each of his or her current mental health/substance abuse supports identified.
9. Individual's strengths and capacities to support good mental health identified.
10. Individual has identified any barriers that are negatively impacting his or her engagement with current mental health/substance supports.
11. Individual has identified any natural supports he or she would like to be involved with in the development of his or her mental health/co-occurring substance abuse supports recovery goal.
12. Individual is aware of crisis-support services in the community and has been provided contact information.
13. Individual is aware of mental health peer support and, as applicable, co-occurring mutual self-help programs in community.

14. Individual has chosen to move forward with his or her mental health and co-occurring supports recovery goal.

___. _____
_____
___. _____
_____
___. _____
_____

Short-term objectives
1. Individual has identified and engaged any natural supports to support his or her mental health and, as applicable, substance abuse recovery goal.
2. Individual is knowledgeable on a range of informal mental health and, as applicable, substance abuse supports available in community.
3. Individual is linked to their desired informal mental health and, as applicable, substance abuse supports available in community.
4. Individual is knowledgeable on a range of formal mental health and, as applicable, substance abuse supports available in community.
5. Individual is linked to their desired formal mental health and, as applicable, substance abuse supports available in community.
6. Individual is engaged and satisfied with mental health/substance abuse supports of choice.

___. _____
_____
___. _____
_____
___. _____
_____

Recovery steps
1. Discuss and inform individual on the range of informal mental health and, as applicable, substance abuse supports and their value (e.g., faith communities; peer support; Compeer Program; self-help groups; Club House Model of Psychosocial Rehabilitation).

2. Discuss with and educate individual on the range of peer support services available in his or her community for mental health and, as applicable, substance abuse supports and their value (e.g., peer counseling/mentoring/coaching; peer mutual aid groups; peer relapse prevention groups; peer conflict resolution skill-building groups; peer advocacy groups; peer telephone support; peer recovery-support drop-in centers; peer support to accompany consumer to treatment services; peer-run alcohol- and substance-free social events).

3. Discuss with and educate individual on the range of self-help groups available in community and their value (e.g., mental health and substance abuse education groups; peer-run groups; veteran self-help groups; online mental health and substance abuse chat groups; stress-management groups; relaxation groups; meditation groups; yoga groups; exercise groups; mindfulness groups; smoking cessation groups; Alcoholic Anonymous; Dual Recovery Anonymous; Double Trouble in Recovery; eating-disorders groups; family support groups; National Alliance for the Mentally Ill groups).

4. Individual identifies any informal mental health and, as applicable, substance abuse supports he or she desires to utilize.

5. Assist individual with linkage to his or her preferred informal mental health/substance abuse supports and accompany him or her to initial linkage if requested.

6. Where individual has requested assistance, obtain signed release of information to speak with any informal supports.

7. If desired, assist individual in discussing with identified natural supports how they can assist individual in achieving his or her mental health/co-occurring substance abuse support goal.

8. Discuss with and inform individual on range of formal mental health and, as applicable, substance abuse and preferably co-occurring supports available in community (e.g., individual therapist—private practice or community mental health; group therapy; integrated co-occurring treatment programs; psycho-education groups; medication management; psychiatric rehabilitation program; PROS—Personalized Recovery Oriented Services; Continuing Day Treatment; Assertive Community Treatment; Intensive Psychiatric Rehabilitation Treatment; Partial Hospitalization; 24-hour crisis line; emergency room).

9. If individual is a veteran, link consumer to Veteran's Administration mental health and, as applicable, substance abuse services as desired.

10. Individual identifies any formal mental health/substance abuse/co-occurring community supports he or she desires to utilize.

11. If individual has both mental health and substance abuse treatment needs, recommend best practice co-occurring integrated treatment if available.

12. If individual is currently engaged in mental health/substance abuse/co-occurring community support services, encourage him or her to discuss desired formal support(s) changes with current providers and if desired, accompany individual.

13. Obtain signed release of information for each preferred formal mental health/substance abuse/co-occurring community support(s) linkage to be made.

14. Link individual to their preferred formal mental health/substance abuse/co-occurring community support(s) and accompany him or her to initial linkage if requested.

15. Assist individual in developing strategies to utilize his or her strengths and capacities to overcome any barriers to achieving his or her mental health /co-occurring substance abuse support recovery goal.

16. Individual discusses levels of participation and satisfaction with mental health/co-occurring substance abuse supports.

17. If individual is not satisfied or engaged in services, offer to meet jointly with the individual and his or her mental health/substance abuse support(s) to assist in resolving any barriers to successful engagement and satisfaction with services.

___. _____

___. _____

___. _____

___. _____

___. _____

LEAVING YOUR PRACTITIONER BEHIND (USING NATURAL ENVIRONMENTS)

Individual's current status
1. Individual is linked to desired natural supports.
2. Individual is linked to desired informal supports.
3. Individual is linked to desired formal supports.
4. Individual is engaged and satisfied with current mental health/co-occurring supports.

___. _____
_____
___. _____
_____
___. _____
_____

Short-term objectives
1. Individual continues engagement and satisfaction with mental health/co-occurring supports.
2. Individual taking primary responsibility for utilizing natural, informal, and formal mental health/substance abuse/co-occurring supports.
3. Individual takes ownership of their mental health/co-occurring substance abuse support recovery goal and has knowledge of where to obtain support if they desire to revise their goal in the future.

___. _____
_____
___. _____
_____
___. _____
_____

Recovery steps
1. Individual shifts focus from direct work to as-needed problem solving with the practitioner on issues that arise with their mental health/co-occurring substance abuse recovery goal.
2. Individual identifies which established natural, informal, and formal supports they wish to continue independently to support good mental health.

3. Individual consults with practitioner as needed.

___. _____
      _____

___. _____
      _____

___. _____
      _____

___. _____
      _____

___. _____
      _____

CHAPTER 4   HOUSING

A housing recovery goal is developed by each individual to assist him or her with securing and retaining a home that is safe, secure, and affordable in support of their recovery.

INDIVIDUAL'S RECOVERY FOCUS

1. Change in housing status.

___. _____

_____

___. _____

_____

BEGINNINGS

Individual's current status
1. Homeless.
2. Inadequate housing.
3. Unstable housing.
4. Nonindependent housing.
5. Stable housing but wants change (e.g., location; size; different landlord).

___. _____

_____

___. _____

_____

Short-term objectives
1. Secure emergency shelter if needed.
2. Individual expresses hopes and dreams regarding housing.
3. Individual provides housing history.
4. Individual identifies his or her strengths and capacities to change housing status.
5. Individual identifies barriers to changing housing status.

6. Individual identifies any natural supports (family/significant others, and/or friends) he or she would like to be involved in their housing recovery goal.
7. Explore with individual housing options in community.
8. Explore with individual peer-support programs in community.
9. Individual expresses housing recovery goal in his or her own words.
10. Individual chooses to move forward on is or her housing recovery goal.

___. _____
    _____
___. _____
    _____
___. _____
    _____

Recovery steps
1. Identify emergency shelter options with individual and link him or her to his or her available choice if needed.
2. Individual explores his or her hopes and dreams regarding housing.
3. Explore how individual sees his or her mental and physical health challenges impacting current housing status.
4. Individual identifies his or her strengths and capacities that can be utilized to overcome barriers and achieve the housing goal.
5. Assist individual in identifying and expressing barriers to his or her housing.
6. Assist individual in identifying and expressing feelings about changing housing status.
7. Individual provides a history of his or her current and previous housing.
8. Determine veteran status.
9. Individual describes current and/or previous successes and challenges in housing environments.
10. Individual identifies any natural supports they would like included in recovery planning meetings.
11. With written permission from the individuals, include identified natural supports in recovery planning meetings as individual desires.

12. Link with any available housing specialist to explore housing and financial support options.
13. Individual identifies risks and benefits to change in housing status.
14. Individual expresses his/her housing recovery goal in his or her own words.
15. Individual chooses to move forward and develop a housing recovery goal.

__. _____
   _____
__. _____
   _____
__. _____
   _____
__. _____
   _____
__. _____
   _____

MOVING FORWARD

Individual's current status

1. Short-term emergency shelter secured as needed.
2. Individual has expressed his or her housing goal in his or her own words.
3. Individual has provided current and previous housing history.
4. Individual's strengths and capacities to support change in housing identified.
5. Individual's barriers to change in housing identified.
6. Individual has determined any natural supports he or she would like to be involved in his or her housing recovery goal.
7. Individual is aware of peer support options in community.
8. Individual is aware of community housing supports.
9. Individual has chosen to move forward on his or her housing recovery goal.

__. _____
   _____
__. _____
   _____

Short-term objectives

1. Individual identifies specific change desired in housing status (i.e., current housing repairs versus different housing).
2. Link individual to community resources to support housing recovery goal.
3. Individual is actively engaged in utilizing linked resources.
4. Increase use of natural supports.
5. Individual is actively implementing housing recovery goal.

__. _____

_____

__. _____

_____

__. _____

_____

Recovery steps

1. Explore with individual the range of housing options available (i.e., independent versus supported living versus staff model support; own versus rent; rooming house versus apartment versus house; consider criminal justice reentry housing programs, as applicable).
2. Discuss availability of housing-support financial assistance available for each housing option.
3. With individual explore his or her view of the pros and cons of each housing option.
4. Assist individual in developing strategies to utilize his or her strengths and capacities to overcome any barriers to achieving his or her self-advocacy goal.
5. Solicit individual's decision about utilizing peer support, and, if the individual is amenable, link to a peer-support agency.
6. Obtain signed release of information to make referral to peer-support agency.
7. If individual chooses a housing support program, refer individual to their program of choice.
8. Obtain signed release of information to make referral to desired housing support program.
9. Refer to veteran-specific housing supports as applicable.
10. If individual chooses not to utilize a housing-support program, explore alternative strategies and resources to support their housing recovery goal as desired.

11. Link individual to their choice of alternative community supports.
12. Link to start-up household furnishings via community programs.
13. Assist individual in obtaining security deposit and/or first month's rent via community programs.
14. Establish regular meetings with individual to support their engagement with established linkages.
15. Encourage ongoing utilization of peer support.
16. Encourage use of natural supports.

—. _____
   _____
—. _____
   _____
—. _____
   _____
—. _____
   _____
—. _____
   _____

LEAVING YOUR PRACTITIONER BEHIND (USING NATURAL ENVIRONMENTS)

Individual's current status
1. Individual is actively implementing housing recovery goal.
2. Individual is linked to community resources to support housing recovery goal.
3. Individual is utilizing strengths and capacities to address barriers to change.
4. Individual is actively engaged in utilizing linked resources.
5. Individual is beginning to use natural supports.

—. _____
   _____
—. _____
   _____

Short-term objectives

1. Individual is taking primary responsibility for moving forward on recovery goal utilizing the support of program linkages, community linkages, and natural supports.
2. Individual takes responsibility for his or her housing recovery goal and has knowledge of where to obtain support if he or she desires to review his or her goal in the future.

___. _____
_____

___. _____
_____

___. _____
_____

Recovery steps

1. Individual shifts focus from direct work to as-needed problem solving with his or her practitioner on the individual's housing recovery goal.
2. Individual identifies which established community linkages and natural supports he or she wishes to continue independently.
3. Individual consults with practitioner as needed.

___. _____
_____

___. _____
_____

___. _____
_____

___. _____
_____

___. _____
_____

CHAPTER 5   EDUCATION

An education recovery goal is developed by the individual to assist him or her with increasing his or her formal learning for personal enrichment as well as to enhance employment opportunities in support of his or her recovery.

INDIVIDUAL'S RECOVERY FOCUS

1. Continue formal education.

___. _____
   _____

___. _____
   _____

BEGINNINGS

Individual's current status
1. Lacks high school diploma.
2. Has high school diploma or GED.
3. Has some college.
4. Desires college degree.

___. _____
   _____

___. _____
   _____

Short-term objectives
1. Individual expresses their hopes and dreams regarding their education.
2. Individual describes past education experience.
3. Individual identifies strengths and capacities to support education.
4. Individual identifies his or her barriers to education.

5. Individual identifies any natural supports (family/significant others and/or friends) he or she might choose to be involved in their education recovery goal.
6. Individual is aware of education opportunities in the community.
7. Individual is aware of peer-support programs in community.
8. Individual expresses willingness to pursue education.

__. _____
   _____
__. _____
   _____
__. _____
   _____

Recovery steps

1. Individual explores his or her hopes and dreams regarding education.
2. Assist individual in identifying and expressing concerns about advancing education.
3. Individual identifies his or her strengths and capacities that can be utilized to overcome barriers and achieve his or her education recovery goal.
4. Assist individual in identifying any barriers to continuing education.
5. Explore how individual sees his or her mental health challenges impacting education.
6. Individual provides his or her education history.
7. Individual describes current and/or previous successes and challenges in educational environments.
8. If individual is a veteran, determine what veteran educational benefits they have used to date.
9. Determine if individual has a documented learning disability.
10. Individual identifies any natural supports they would like included in his or her recovery-goal planning meetings.
11. With written permission from the individuals, include identified natural supports in recovery-goal planning meetings as individual desires.
12. Individual provided information on the value of working with a peer-support program.
13. Individual identifies risks and benefits to continuing education.

14. Explore with individual the kinds and scope of educational programs that are available to individual in the community.
15. Individual expresses his or her education goal in his or her own words.
16. Individual chooses to move forward with his or her education recovery goal.

—. _____
   _____
—. _____
   _____
—. _____
   _____
—. _____
   _____
—. _____
   _____

MOVING FORWARD

Individual's current status

1. Individual has expressed the education goal in his or her own words.
2. Individual's strengths and capacities to support education are identified.
3. Individual's barriers to education are identified.
4. Individual has chosen any natural supports he or she would like to be involved in the individual's education recovery goal.
5. Individual is aware of community education opportunities.
6. Individual is aware of peer-support programs in community.
7. Individual has chosen to move forward on his or her education recovery goal.

—. _____
   _____
—. _____
   _____

Short-term objectives

1. Individual identifies specific education goal.

2. Individual is linked to informal and formal community resources to support education recovery goal.
3. Individual is actively engaged in utilizing linked resources.
4. Individual is increasing use of preferred natural supports.
5. Individual is actively implementing education recovery goal.

—. _____

_____

—. _____

_____

—. _____

_____

Recovery steps
1. Identify with individual education programs of interest available in community.
2. Encourage individual to explore online educational programs of interest to him or her.
3. Assist individual with determining where there is computer access in the community that he or she can utilize.
4. Encourage individual to personally visit educational programs of interest and offer to accompany him or her, should individual choose.
5. Discuss individual's view of the pros and cons of each education program.
6. Assist individual in developing strategies to utilize his or her strengths and capacities to overcome any barriers to achieving his or her education recovery goal.
7. Explore with individual any educational support options that may be available.
8. Refer to veteran educational supports as applicable.
9. Solicit individual's decision about utilizing peer support, and if individual is amenable to support, link to a peer-support agency.
10. Obtain signed release of information to make referral to peer-support agency.
11. Support individual in contacting education program of choice and navigating admission process.
12. Support individual in identifying financial aid options for education program of choice and application process.

13. Support individual in exploring disability supports as available in education program of choice and, if agreed, support enrollment in same.
14. Establish regular meetings with individual to support his or her engagement with established linkages.
15. Encourage ongoing utilization of peer support.
16. Encourage use of natural supports.

___. _____
      _____
___. _____
      _____
___. _____
      _____
___. _____
      _____
___. _____
      _____

LEAVING YOUR PRACTITIONER BEHIND (USING NATURAL ENVIRONMENTS)

Individual's current status
1. Individual is utilizing his or her strengths to address barriers to change.
2. Individual is actively implementing education recovery goal.
3. Individual is linked to informal and formal community resources to support education recovery goal.
4. Individual is actively engaged in utilizing linked resources.
6. Individual is beginning to use natural supports.

___. _____
      _____
___. _____
      _____

Short-term objectives
1. Individual taking primary responsibility for moving forward on recovery goal utilizing the support of community linkages and natural supports.

2. Individual takes primary responsibility for his or her education recovery goal and has knowledge about where to obtain support if individual desires to revise his or her goal in the future.

___. _____
_____

___. _____
_____

___. _____
_____

Recovery steps

1. Individual shifts focus from direct work to as-needed problem solving with the practitioner on the individual's education recovery goal.
2. Individual identifies which established community linkages and natural supports he or she wishes to continue independently.
3. Individual consults with practitioner as needed.

___. _____
_____

___. _____
_____

___. _____
_____

___. _____
_____

___. _____
_____

CHAPTER 6   LEGAL

A legal recovery goal is developed by the individual to assist him or her with acquiring the knowledge and resources necessary to resolve his or her legal challenges and move forward in support of his or her recovery.

INDIVIDUAL'S RECOVERY FOCUS

1. Resolve legal issues.

___. _____
_____
___. _____
_____

BEGINNINGS

Individual's current status
1. Legal issue pending.
2. Needs to follow legal/court requirements/recommendations.
3. Needs to meet probation requirements.
4. Need to meet parole requirements.

___. _____
_____
___. _____
_____

Short-term objectives
1. Individual expresses hopes and dreams regarding legal goal.
2. Individual provides history of legal issues.
3. Individual secures legal counsel as needed.
4. Individual's eligibility determined for mental health and drug court as available and appropriate to needs.
5. With individual, identify his or her strengths and capacities to support achieving his or her legal goal.

6. With individual, identify barriers to achieving individual's legal goal.
7. Individual identifies any natural supports (family/significant others and/or friends) he or she would like to be involved in his or her legal recovery goal.
8. Educate on legal supports in community.
9. Explore with individual peer-support programs in community.
10. Individual expresses his or her legal recovery goal in his or her own words.
11. Individual chooses to move forward with his or her legal recovery goal.

—. _____
_____
—. _____
_____
—. _____
_____

Recovery steps

1. Explore with individual his or her hopes and dreams regarding his or her legal goal.
2. Individual provides history related to current legal issue, including arrests, cases pending, convictions, current legal requirements including probation and parole.
3. Assist individual in identifying and expressing concerns about current legal status.
4. Individual identifies his or her strengths and capacities that can be utilized to reduce concerns and achieve legal recovery goal.
5. Explore with individual how he or she sees their mental health challenges impacting current legal status.
6. As applicable, explore with individual how substance use is impacting his or her current legal status.
7. Determine veteran status.
8. With individual, explore legal and, as applicable, reentry resources in community.
9. Link with legal counsel as needed and desired (e.g., public defender; Legal Aid Bureau; private attorney including pro bono).

10. With individual's permission, explore with individual and his or her legal counsel the appropriateness and availability of transferring any pending case to Mental Health Court, if applicable.

11. With individual's permission, explore with individual and his or her legal counsel the appropriateness and availability of transferring any pending case to Drug Court, if applicable.

12. If individual is a veteran, and with individual's permission, explore with individual and his or her legal counsel the appropriateness and availability of transferring any pending case to Veteran's Court.

13. Individual explores any barriers to achieving his or her legal goal.

14. Individual identifies any natural supports he or she would like included in his or her recovery planning meetings.

15. With written permission, include identified natural supports in recovery-goal planning meetings as individual desires.

16. Explore with individual peer-support programs in community.

17. Individual expresses his/her legal recovery goal in his or her own words.

18. Individual chooses to move forward on his or her legal recovery goal.

__. _____
     _____
__. _____
     _____
__. _____
     _____
__. _____
     _____
__. _____
     _____

MOVING FORWARD

Individual's current status

1. Individual has expressed in his/her own words his or her legal recovery goal.

2. Individual has provided legal history of current legal issue.

3. Individual has secured legal counsel as needed.

4. Individual's eligibility determined for Mental Health, Drug, and Veteran's Court as available and appropriate to needs.

5. Individual's strengths and capacities to support achieving his or her legal goal have been identified.
6. Individual's barriers to achieving his or her legal goal has been identified.
7. Natural supports the individual would like to be involved in their legal recovery goal have been identified.
8. Individual is aware of legal and reentry supports in community.
9. Individual is aware of peer-support programs in community.
10. Individual chooses to move forward on his or her legal recovery goal.

—. _____
   _____
—. _____
   _____

Short-term objectives
1. Individual is linked to desired resources to address his or her legal recovery goal.
2. Individual is aware of any probation or parole requirements and has identified any challenges to meeting requirements.
3. Individual linked to legal, reentry supports, and formally incarcerated person supports.
4. Individual is linked to peer-support programs.
5. Individual is actively engaged in utilizing linked formal and informal resources.
6. Individual is increasing use of natural supports.
7. Individual is actively implementing legal recovery goal.

—. _____
   _____
—. _____
   _____
—. _____
   _____

Recovery steps
1. Individual describes his or her probation requirements (e.g., curfew; job requirements; drug testing; living restrictions; restitution) as applicable.

2. Individual reviews each probation requirement and identifies any related challenges to meeting them.

3. Assist individual in problem-solving probation requirement challenges and assist the individual in developing his or her plan to address each.

4. Individual describes his or her parole requirements (e.g., curfew; job requirements; drug testing; living restrictions; restitution) as applicable.

5. Individual reviews each parole requirement and identifies any related challenges to meeting each.

6. Assist individual in problem-solving parole-requirement challenges and assist individual in developing his or her plan to address each.

7. Explore with individual range of support groups and programs in the community (e.g., reentry support group; faith-based ministries support program; ex-offenders support group; job programs for ex-offenders; Urban League support programs; veteran support group).

8. Link individual to support groups and programs of his or her choice and offer to accompany him or her to first meeting(s).

9. If substance abuse is identified, discuss with individual if they are currently in a co-occurring treatment program; if not and individual is agreeable, link individual to same.

10. Solicit individual's decision about utilizing peer support, and if so, link to peer-support programs (e.g., peer counseling/mentoring/coaching; peer-run support groups; peer-advocacy services).

11. Obtain signed release of information to make referral to peer-support agency.

12. Assist individual in developing strategies to utilize his or her strengths and capacities to overcome any barriers to achieving his or her legal recovery goal.

13. Establish regular meetings with individual to support their active engagement with established linkages.

14. Encourage ongoing utilization of peer support.

15. Encourage use of natural supports.

—. _____
   _____
—. _____
   _____

—. _____
   _____
—. _____
   _____
   _____
—. _____
   _____

LEAVING YOUR PRACTITIONER BEHIND (USING NATURAL ENVIRONMENTS)

Individual's current status

1. Actively implementing legal recovery goal.
2. Linked to community resources to support legal recovery goal.
3. Individual is utilizing strengths and capacities to support legal recovery goal.
4. Individual is beginning to use natural supports.
5. Actively engaged in utilizing linked resources.

—. _____
   _____
—. _____
   _____
   _____
—. _____
   _____

Short-term objectives

1. Individual continues engagement and satisfaction with legal goal supports.
2. Individual taking primary responsibility for utilizing legal, natural, and peer supports.
3. Individual takes ownership of his or her legal recovery goal and has knowledge about where to obtain support if he or she desires to revise the goal in the future.

—. _____
   _____
—. _____
   _____
   _____
—. _____
   _____

Recovery steps

1. Individual shifts focus from direct work to as-needed problem solving with the practitioner on issues that arise with his or her legal recovery goal.
2. Individual identifies which legal, natural, and peer supports he or she wishes to continue independently to support his or her legal recovery goal.
3. Individual consults with practitioner as needed.

___. _____

    _____

___. _____

    _____

___. _____

    _____

___. _____

    _____

___. _____

    _____

CHAPTER 7   EMPLOYMENT

An employment recovery goal is developed by the individual to assist him or her with obtaining his or her desired employment in the community in support of the individual's recovery.

INDIVIDUAL'S RECOVERY FOCUS

1. Change in employment status.

__. _____
    _____
__. _____
    _____

BEGINNINGS

Individual's current status
1. Unemployed.
2. Underemployed.
3. Never employed.
4. Desires change in employment.

__. _____
    _____
__. _____
    _____

Short-term objectives
1. Individual expresses his or her hopes and dreams regarding employment.
2. Individual provides history of employment, education, and/or skills and training.
3. Individual identifies strengths and capacities to support employment.
4. Individual's barriers to employment are identified.

5. Individual identifies any natural supports (family/significant others and/or friends) they would like to be involved in his or her employment recovery goal.
6. Individual is aware of vocational-support programs in community.
7. Individual is aware of peer-support programs in community.
8. Individual has expressed his or her employment recovery goal in his or her own words.
9. Individual has chosen to move forward on his or her employment recovery goal.

—. _____

   _____

   _____

—. _____

   _____

—. _____

   _____

Recovery steps
1. Explore individual's hopes and dreams regarding employment.
2. Assist individual in identifying and expressing his or her concerns about changing employment status.
3. Explore how individual sees his or her mental health challenges impacting employment.
4. Individual identifies his or her strengths and capacities that can be utilized to achieve employment recovery goal.
5. Assist individual in identifying barriers to employment.
6. Individual provides his or her employment, education, and/or training skills history.
7. Individual describes current and/or previous successes and challenges in work environments.
8. Individual identifies any natural supports they would like included in his or her employment recovery-goal planning meetings.
9. With written permission from the individual, include identified natural supports recovery-goal planning meetings as consumer desires.
10. Explore with individual the value of working with a peer-support agency.
11. Individual signs a release for referral to a peer-support agency.

12. Link with benefits specialist to increase awareness of how a change of employment status impacts benefits (e.g., SSI, SSD, Medicaid).
13. Individual identifies risks and benefits to employment.
14. Explore with individual the kinds and scope of vocational programs they may be interested in and/or eligible for in community.
15. Individual has expressed his or her recovery goal in his or her own words.
16. Individual chooses to move forward on his or her employment recovery goal.

—. _____
    _____
—. _____
    _____
—. _____
    _____
—. _____
    _____
—. _____
    _____

MOVING FORWARD

Individual's current status:
1. Individual has expressed his or her employment recovery goal in his or her own words.
2. Individual has provided a history of his or her employment, education, and/or training skills.
3. Individual strengths and capacities to support employment identified.
4. Individual barriers to employment identified.
5. Individual is aware of community vocational supports.
6. Individual is aware of peer-support programs in community.
7. Individual has chosen to move forward on his or her employment recovery goal.

—. _____
    _____
—. _____
    _____

Short-term objectives

1. Individual identifies specific change desired in employment status.
2. Link individual to informal and formal community resources to support employment recovery goal.
3. Individual is actively engaged in utilizing linked resources.
4. Individual is increasing use of natural supports.
5. Individual is actively implementing employment recovery goal.

—. _____
_____

—. _____
_____

—. _____
_____

Recovery steps

1. Explore employment options with individual.
2. Discuss individual's view of the pros and cons of each employment option.
3. Identify formal education needed for specific employment choices.
4. Develop with individual educational goal within his or her recovery plan to support employment goal.
5. Solicit individual's decision about utilizing peer support, and if individual is amenable, link to a peer-support agency.
6. Obtain signed release of information to make referral to peer-support agency.
7. Review with individual community vocational-support program options.
8. Solicit individual's decision about utilizing a vocational-support program, and if the individual is amenable, refer to individual's program of choice.
9. If individual chooses not to utilize a vocational program, explore alternative strategies and resources to support individual's employment recovery goal.
10. Obtain a signed release of information for referral to vocational-support program or as needed for any alternative community supports.
11. Link to preferred vocational-support program or alternative community supports.

12. Assist individual in developing strategies to utilize his or her strengths and capacities to overcome any barriers to achieving his or her employment recovery goal.
13. Assist individual in resume development.
14. Discuss with individual appropriate interview apparel and link as necessary to clothing closet.
15. Role-play mock interview.
16. Establish regular meetings with individual to support his or her engagement with established linkages.
17. Encourage ongoing utilization of peer support.
18. Encourage use of natural supports.

—. _____
   _____
   _____
—. _____
   _____
   _____
—. _____
   _____
   _____
—. _____
   _____
   _____
—. _____
   _____

LEAVING YOUR PRACTITIONER BEHIND (USING NATURAL ENVIRONMENTS)

Individual's current status
1. Individual is actively implementing employment recovery goal.
2. Individual is linked to informal and formal community resources to support employment recovery goal.
3. Individual is beginning to use natural supports.
4. Individual is actively engaged in utilizing linked resources.

—. _____
   _____
   _____
—. _____
   _____

Short-term objectives

1. Individual taking primary responsibility for moving forward on employment recovery goal utilizing the support of community linkages and natural supports.
2. Individual takes responsibility for his or her employment recovery goal and has the knowledge of where to obtain support if they desire to revise his or her goal in the future.

___. _____
   _____
___. _____
   _____
___. _____
   _____

Recovery steps

1. Individual shifts focus from direct work to as-needed problem solving with practitioner about his or her employment recovery goal.
2. Individual identifies which established community linkages and natural supports he or she wishes to continue independently to support his or her employment recovery goal.
3. Individual consults with practitioner as needed.

___. _____
   _____
___. _____
   _____
___. _____
   _____
___. _____
   _____
___. _____
   _____

CHAPTER 8   FINANCIAL STABILITY

A financial stability recovery goal is developed by the individual to promote financial knowledge and empower the individual to maximize his or her financial resources in support of his or her recovery.

INDIVIDUAL'S RECOVERY FOCUS

1. Maximize resources to support financial stability goal.

__. _____

   _____

__. _____

   _____

BEGINNINGS

Individual's current status

1. No source of income.
2. Inadequate income.
3. Desire to improve financial stability.
4. Financial crisis.

__. _____

   _____

__. _____

   _____

Short-term objectives

1. Individual expresses his or her hopes and dreams regarding finances.
2. Individual provides his or her financial history and current financial resources.
3. With individual, determine his or her monthly living expenses.
4. Individual identifies his or her strengths and capacities to support improving financial stability.

5. Individual identifies barriers to improving his or her financial stability.
6. Individual identifies any natural supports (family/significant others and/or friends) they would like to be involved in his or her financial stability recovery goal.
7. With individual, explore the range of community resources the individual may be eligible for.
8. With individual, explore peer-support programs in community.
9. Individual expresses his or her financial stability goal in his or her own words.
10. Individual chooses to move forward on his or her financial stability goal.

—. _____

_____

—. _____

_____

—. _____

_____

Recovery steps
1. Explore with individual his or her immediate basic needs (e.g., food, shelter).
2. Link individual to emergency support services (i.e., social services, Salvation Army; Catholic Charities) if needed.
3. Individual explores his or her hopes and dreams regarding financial stability.
4. Explore with individual how they see his or her mental health challenges impacting his or her financial stability.
5. Assist in identifying and expressing concerns about achieving financial stability.
6. Individual identifies risks and benefits to financial stability.
7. Individual identifies his or her strengths and capacities that can be utilized to reduce barriers to achieving his or her financial recovery goal.
8. Individual identifies barriers to achieving financial stability.
9. With individual, determine his or her current sources of income (e.g., employment; child support; SSI; SSD).

10. With individual, determine current community supports they utilize (e.g., bank; food pantry; coupon clipping group; soup kitchen).
11. With individual, determine his or her monthly living expenses.
12. Explore with individual his or her history of managing finances.
13. Individual describes current and/or previous successes and challenges managing finances.
14. Individual identifies any natural supports they would like included in recovery-goal planning meetings.
15. With written permission from the individual, include identified natural supports in recovery-goal planning meetings, as individual desires.
16. Explore with individual the range and types of resources available in the community.
17. Explore with individual the value of working with a peer-support agency.
18. Individual expresses his or her financial stability goal in his or her own words.
19. Individual chooses to move forward on his or her financial stability goal.

—. _____

—. _____
_____

—. _____
_____

—. _____
_____

—. _____
_____

MOVING FORWARD

Individual's current status

1. Individual's immediate emergency needs met, if needed.
2. Individual has expressed his or her financial stability goal in his or her own words.
3. Financial history and current financial resources determined.
4. Individual's current living expenses determined.

5. Individual has identified his or her strengths and capacities to support financial stability identified.
6. Individual has identified barriers to financial stability.
7. Individual is aware of range of community resources available, which they may be eligible for.
8. Individual is aware of peer-support programs in community.
9. Individual has chosen to move forward on his or her financial stability goal.

____. _____
       _____
____. _____
       _____

Short-term objectives
1. Individual identifies specific change(s) to achieve financial stability goal.
2. Link individual to community resources to support financial recovery goal.
3. Individual is actively engaged in utilizing linked resources.
4. Individual is increasing use of natural supports.
5. Individual is actively implementing his or her financial recovery goal.

____. _____
       _____
____. _____
       _____
____. _____
       _____

Recovery steps
1. Review with individual his or her monthly living expenses and income.
2. Determine causal factor(s) driving the income/expense difference.
3. Determine, with individual, difference between income and expenses.
4. Assist individual in developing budget for living expenses.
5. Assist individual in developing strategies to utilize his or her strengths and capacities to overcome any obstacles to achieving his or her financial stability goal.

6. Explore, with individual, his or her view of the costs and benefits of improving his or her financial stability.
7. Assist individual in developing strategies to utilize his or her strengths and capacities to overcome any obstacles to achieving his or her financial stability goal.
8. Determine veteran status.
9. If veteran, link to a veteran's benefit specialist, if desired.
10. Link to Social Services to determine eligibility for public assistance and assist individual as appropriate with the application process (e.g., food stamps, heat assistance).
11. Link to Social Security, and assist individual, as appropriate, with application process for SSI and/or SSD.
12. Assist individual with learning about representative payee services and, if appropriate and agreed, assist in application process.
13. Provide individual with list of local food pantries, soup kitchens, and clothes closets.
14. Link to not-for-profit Financial Counseling Services to explore reduction of outstanding debt.
15. If individual is a parent and not receiving child support, link to Child Support Collection Unit and/or Neighborhood Legal Services.
16. Assist in application process for student loan forgiveness if individual has a permanent disability.
17. Link to money management support/education group.
18. Link to benefit specialist.
19. Link to subsidized housing programs to determine eligibility/availability (e.g., Supportive Housing, Section 8).
20. Identify formal education needed for any specific employment choices.
21. Solicit individual's decision about utilizing peer support.
22. Obtain signed release of information to make referral to peer-support agency as indicated.
23. Review community vocational-support program options.
24. Establish regular meetings with individual to support his or her engagement with established linkages.
25. Encourage ongoing utilization of peer support.
26. Encourage use of natural supports.

—. _____
   _____
—. _____

_____. _____

_____. _____

_____. _____

LEAVING YOUR PRACTITIONER BEHIND (USING NATURAL ENVIRONMENTS)

Individual's current status

1. Individual is actively implementing financial recovery goal.
2. Individual is linked to community resources and natural supports to support financial recovery goal.
3. Individual is beginning to use natural supports.
4. Individual is actively engaged in utilizing linked resources.

_____. _____

_____. _____

Short-term objectives

1. Individual continues engagement and satisfaction with financial stability goal.
2. Individual taking primary responsibility for moving forward on recovery goal, utilizing the support of community linkages and natural supports.
3. Individual takes ownership of his or her financial stability goal and has knowledge of where to obtain support if he or she desires to revise his or her goal in the future.

_____. _____

_____. _____

_____. _____

Recovery steps

1. Individual shifts focus from direct work to as-needed problem solving with the practitioner on his or her financial stability recovery goal.
2. Individual identifies which established community linkages and natural supports he or she wishes to continue independently.
3. Individual consults with practitioner as needed.

___. _____

___. _____

___. _____

___. _____

___. _____

CHAPTER 9   SELF-ADVOCACY

A self-advocacy recovery goal is developed by the individual to assist the individual with increasing and/or improving his or her self-advocacy skills to empower the individual to positively influence persons, programs, organizations, policies, and more to support the individual's recovery.

INDIVIDUAL'S RECOVERY FOCUS

1. Increase and/or improve self-advocacy skills.

__. _____
    _____

__. _____
    _____

BEGINNINGS

Individual's current status
1. Dissatisfied with current self-advocacy skills.
2. Minimal knowledge of rights.
3. Low self-esteem/self-confidence.
4. Desire to increase self-advocacy skills.

__. _____
    _____

__. _____
    _____

Short-term objectives
1. Individual is knowledgeable about self-advocacy and its value to promoting the individual's own recovery.
2. Individual expresses his or her hopes and dreams regarding self-advocacy skills.

3. Individual is aware of the range of life areas in which self-advocacy skills would be helpful (e.g., friends; family; significant other; neighbors; landlord; mental health providers; social service agencies; bill collectors; car repair companies; employers).
4. Individual identifies his or her strengths and capacities to support self-advocacy recovery goal.
5. Individual identifies barriers to self-advocacy.
6. Individual identifies any natural supports (family/significant others and/or friends) they wish to include in recovery-goal planning meetings.
7. Individual expresses his or her self-advocacy recovery goal in his or her own words.
8. Individual chooses to move forward on his or her self-advocacy recovery goal.

___. _____
    _____
___. _____
    _____
___. _____
    _____

Recovery steps
1. With individual, discuss what self-advocacy is and its value to promoting his or her own recovery.
2. Explore with individual the areas of his or her life where self-advocacy skills might be helpful (e.g., friends; family; significant other; neighbors; landlord; mental health providers; social service agencies; bill collectors; car repair company; employer).
3. With individual explore his or her hopes and dreams regarding self-advocacy skills.
4. Individual explores the challenges and benefits to improving his or her self-advocacy skills.
5. Individual identifies how mental health challenges have impacted his or her ability to self-advocate.
6. Individual expresses how self-advocacy may improve his or her quality of life.
7. Increase awareness of how self-advocacy, or the lack thereof, may promote or hinder recovery.

8. Individual identifies his or her strengths and capacities that can be utilized to support his or her self-advocacy goal.
9. Individual identifies any barriers to achieving his or her self-advocacy recovery goal.
10. With individual, identify any natural supports they would like included in development of his or her self-advocacy recovery goal.
11. With written permission from the individual, include natural supports identified in recovery-goal planning meetings, as individual desires.
12. Explore with individual peer-support programs in community.
13. Individual expresses his or her self-advocacy-skills recovery goal in his or her own words.
14. Individual chooses to move forward and implement his or her self-advocacy recovery goal.

—. _____
 _____
 _____
—. _____
 _____
 _____
—. _____
 _____
 _____
—. _____
 _____
 _____
—. _____
 _____

MOVING FORWARD

Individual's current status:
1. Individual has expressed his or her self-advocacy recovery goal in his or her own words.
2. Individual is aware of the range of life areas where self-advocacy skills would be helpful.
3. Individual's strengths and capacities to support self-advocacy recovery goal have been identified.
4. Individual's barriers to self-advocacy identified.
5. Individual has identified any natural supports he or she wishes to include in recovery-goal planning meetings.
6. Individual has chosen to move forward and implement his or her self-advocacy recovery goal.

—. _____
    _____
—. _____
    _____
—. _____
    _____

Short-term objectives

1. Explore with individual self-advocacy strategies.
2. Explore with individual the full range of self-advocacy skill-building opportunities and supports.
3. Link individual to his or her preferred informal and formal self-advocacy skills-building resources.
4. Increase use of natural supports.

—. _____
    _____
—. _____
    _____
—. _____
    _____

Recovery steps

1. Link individual to educational resources to promote self-advocacy knowledge and skills (e.g., library; online resources; community education classes; peer-run advocacy organizations; Legal Aid; college classes; local politician's offices; Mental Health Association advocacy supports).
2. Assist individual in developing strategies to utilize his or her strengths and capacities to overcome any barriers to achieving his or her self-advocacy goal.
3. Individual identifies current self-advocacy priorities.
4. Individual identifies persons/organizations they need to influence to achieve his or her self-advocacy priorities.
5. Support individual in identifying his or her potential approaches to advocating for the change they desire (e.g., in-person meeting; writing a letter; sending e-mail or letter to the editor; involving a peer or peer organization in supporting his or her efforts; obtaining legal counsel).

6. Identify with individual effective self-advocacy communication skills (e.g., verbally and/or in writing articulate clearly what they want changed; conflict-resolution skills such as asserting oneself respectfully and remaining calm in the face of opposition).

7. Role-play with individual advocating for one or more of his or her identified priorities for desired change, utilizing effective communication skills.

8. Encourage individual to practice his or her self-advocacy skills with identified natural supports.

9. Identify with individual informal self-advocacy skills-building opportunities and supports in the community (e.g., community education programs; faith-based programs; self-help groups; YouTube self-advocacy skills training videos).

10. Identify with individual the range of peer support self-advocacy skills-building opportunities and supports in the community (e.g., peer counseling/mentoring/coaching; peer-run advocacy-training classes; peer-run self-esteem group; peer-run support group; peer-run communication-skills group; peer-run assertiveness group).

11. Individual identifies any informal self-advocacy skills-building opportunities and supports they desire to utilize.

12. Assist individual with linkage to his or her preferred informal self-advocacy building opportunities and supports and accompany them to initial linkage if desired.

13. Where individual has requested assistance, obtain signed release of information to speak with any informal supports.

14. Identify with individual the range of formal social skills–building opportunities and supports available in community (e.g., individual therapist—private practice or community mental health; care coordinator; communication skills–building group; self-esteem group; assertiveness training group; psycho-education groups; psychiatric rehabilitation program; PROS—Personalized Recovery Oriented Services; Continuing Day Treatment; Intensive Psychiatric Rehabilitation Treatment).

15. If individual is a veteran, link to Veteran Administration for self-advocacy building opportunities and supports, as available and desired.

16. Individual identifies any formal self-advocacy opportunities and supports they desire to utilize.

17. Obtain signed release of information to facilitate linkage to formal self-advocacy skills opportunities and supports.

18. Assist individual with linkage to his or her preferred formal self-advocacy skills-building opportunities and supports and accompany them to initial linkage if desired.
19. Support individual in identifying any required financial costs for linkages, and problem-solve funding needs as necessary.
20. Support individual in identifying any transportation barriers and problem solve as needed
21. Establish regular meetings with individual to support his or her engagement with established linkages.
22. Encourage ongoing use of peer support.

___. _____
    _____
___. _____
    _____
___. _____
    _____
___. _____
    _____
___. _____
    _____

LEAVING YOUR PRACTITIONER BEHIND (USING NATURAL ENVIRONMENTS)

Individual's status
1. Individual is linked to desired informal supports.
2. Individual is linked to desired formal supports.
3. Individual is beginning to use natural supports.
4. Individual is engaged and satisfied with current self-advocacy recovery-goal linkages.

___. _____
    _____
___. _____
    _____
___. _____
    _____

Short-term objectives

1. Individual maintains engagement and satisfaction with self-advocacy skills-building opportunities and supports.
2. Individual takes primary responsibility for utilizing natural, informal, and formal self-advocacy skills-building opportunities and supports.
3. Individual takes responsibility for his or her self-advocacy recovery goal and has knowledge of where to obtain support if he or she desires to revise his or her goal in the future.

—. _____

_____

—. _____

_____

—. _____

_____

Recovery steps

1. Individual shifts focus from direct work to as-needed problem solving with his or her practitioner about his or her self-advocacy recovery goal.
2. Individual identifies which established natural, informal, and formal supports they wish to continue independently to support his or her self-advocacy recovery goal.
3. Individual consults practitioner as needed.

—. _____

_____

—. _____

_____

—. _____

_____

—. _____

_____

—. _____

_____

CHAPTER 10   FAMILY RELATIONSHIPS

A family-relationships recovery goal is developed by the individual to assist him or her with reengaging, enhancing, and/or restructuring desired family relationships in support of the individual's recovery.

INDIVIDUAL'S RECOVERY FOCUS

1. Change relationship with family.

__. _____
_____

__. _____
_____

BEGINNINGS

Individual's current status

1. Dependent on family.
2. Estranged from family.
3. Family conflict.
4. Family overinvolvement.
5. Family underinvolvement.

__. _____
_____

__. _____
_____

Short-term objectives

1. Determine who individual identifies as his or her family.
2. Understand current relationship with family.
3. Identify significant family member(s) for relationship change.
4. Determine relationship change desired.
5. Individual strengths to support change identified.
6. Barriers to family relationship change identified.

7. Individual expresses family relationships goal in his or her own words.
8. Individual chooses to move forward on his or her family relationships goal.

___. _____
_____

___. _____
_____

___. _____
_____

Recovery steps

1. Individual explores his or her hopes and dreams regarding his or her family relationships.
2. Individual identifies his or her significant family members.
3. Individual describes history of relationship(s) with identified family members.
4. Individual identifies how mental health challenges have impacted family relationship.
5. Explore how individual sees how change in family relationships may improve his or her quality of life.
6. Assist individual defining and expressing change desired.
7. Increase awareness of family role in promoting or hindering recovery.
8. Individual identifies his or her strengths and capacities that can be utilized to achieve family relationships recovery goal.
9. Individual identifies barriers to achieving desired family relationship change.
10. Individual identifies any risks and benefits to desired change.
11. Identify with individual any natural supports (family/significant others and/or friends) they would like included in recovery planning meetings.
12. With written permission from the individual, include identified natural supports in recovery planning meetings as individual desires.
13. Individual expresses his or her family-relationships goal in his or her own words.

14. Individual chooses to move forward with his or her family relationships goal.

___. _____
    _____
    _____
___. _____
    _____
    _____
___. _____
    _____
    _____
___. _____
    _____
    _____
___. _____
    _____
    _____

MOVING FORWARD

Individual's current status

1. Individual has expressed his or her family relationships goal in his or her own words.
2. Individual has defined who his or her family is.
3. Current relationship with family determined.
4. Individual expresses relationship change desired.
5. Significant family member(s) for relationship change identified.
6. Individual's strengths and capacities identified to support change.
7. Barriers to change family relationships identified.
8. Individual has identified any natural supports he or she wishes to include in recovery-goal planning meetings.
9. Individual has chosen to move forward on his or her family relation-ships goal.

___. _____
    _____
    _____
___. _____
    _____
    _____
___. _____
    _____
    _____

Short-term objectives

1. Significant family member(s) engaged to participate in individual's family relationships recovery goal.

2. Identify family strengths and capacities for achieving change.
3. Identify family barriers to changing relationship.
4. Individual and family identify supports to effect change.
5. Increase family knowledge of mental health and any co-occurring substance abuse challenges and recovery.
6. Improve family relationship.

—. _____

_____

—. _____

_____

—. _____

_____

Recovery steps

1. Assist individual in locating family member(s).
2. Support individual contacting family.
3. Rehearse with individual expressing his or her goal directly with family.
4. Arrange family meeting, including individual to discuss role of family in recovery and individual's family relationships recovery goal.
5. Individual expresses goal directly with family.
6. Explore family member's hopes and concerns together with individual regarding relationship with individual.
7. Assess family member's willingness to engage/reengage with individual and at what level.
8. Assist individual and family member(s) in identifying family strengths and capacities to support change.
9. Assist individual and family member(s) in identifying any barriers to changing relationship.
10. Assist individual in developing strategies to utilize his or her strengths and capacities to overcome any barriers to achieving his or her family relationships goal.
11. Discuss with individual and family the value of peer support.
12. Include a peer advocate in family meeting(s) as individual desires and family agrees.
13. Support family meetings and provide conflict resolution as necessary.
14. Refer family member(s) to psycho-education family group.

15. Discuss with individual and family how family strengths and capacities will be utilized to support desired change.
16. Provide referral for family therapy as indicated and desired.
17. Introduce and discuss the value of the National Alliance on Mental Illness (NAMI) as a possible resource with individual and family.
18. Link individual and family to NAMI as desired.
19. Assess need for respite care with family and individual.
20. Identify respite resources and link individual and family as needed and desired.
21. Link family members to social service supports where indicated and desired.
22. Arrange transportation for individual as needed to support family relationships recovery goal.
23. Problem-solve with family any transportation barriers they may have to supporting individual's family relationships recovery goal.
24. Link family to support group, if desired.
25. Link to relationship-skill building group.
26. Provide education to family member(s) on mental health challenges and any co-occurring substance abuse concerns and its impact on both the individual and the family.
27. Refer family member(s) to a stress-reduction group if indicated and desired.

—. _____
   _____
—. _____
   _____
—. _____
   _____
—. _____
   _____
—. _____
   _____

LEAVING YOUR PRACTITIONER BEHIND (USING NATURAL ENVIRONMENTS)

Individual's current status

1. Significant family member(s) engaged and participating with individual in family relationships recovery goal.

2. Individual and family are utilizing his or her strengths to address any barriers to change.
3. Individual and family are utilizing natural, informal, and formal supports to effect change identified.
4. Individual and family are more knowledgeable of mental health challenges and any co-occurring substance abuse concerns and its impact on relationships and recovery.
5. Family relationship(s) improving.

___. _____

_____

___. _____

_____

___. _____

_____

Short-term objectives

1. Individual identifies which established natural, informal, and formal supports they wish to continue independently to support his or her family relationships recovery goal.
2. Individual takes responsibility for his or her family relationships recovery goal and has knowledge of where to obtain support if he or she desires to revise his or her goal in the future.

___. _____

_____

___. _____

_____

___. _____

_____

Recovery steps

1. Individual shifts focus from direct work to as-needed problem solving with the practitioner, his or her community linkages, and natural supports.
2. Individual identifies which natural, informal, and formal supports he or she wishes to continue independently to support his or her family relationships recovery goal.
3. Sustain NAMI as a resource if desired.

4. Individual consults with practitioner as needed.

___. _____
_____

___. _____
_____

___. _____
_____

___. _____
_____

___. _____
_____

CHAPTER 11   HEALTH AND WELLNESS

A health and wellness recovery goal is developed by the individual to empower him or her to maximize his or her own health and wellness in support of his or her recovery.

INDIVIDUAL'S RECOVERY FOCUS

1.   Improve health and wellness.

___. _____

_____

___. _____

_____

BEGINNINGS

Individual's current status

1.   Poor health and wellness.
2.   Marginal health and wellness.
3.   Maintain health and wellness.

___. _____

_____

___. _____

_____

Short-term objectives

1.   Individual identifies his or her hopes and dreams regarding his or her health and wellness.
2.   Introduce individual to dimensions of wellness including physical, intellecttual, emotional, social, spiritual, environmental, and occupational.
3.   Individual prioritizes one or more dimensions of health they choose to work on.
4.   Explore how individual has historically dealt with health and wellness.

5. Identify how individual currently engages in health and wellness activities and strategies.
6. Individual identifies his or her strengths and capacities to improve or change health and wellness.
7. Individual identifies current barriers to health and wellness.
8. Identify with individual natural supports (family/significant others and/or friends) he or she would like to be involved in his or her health and wellness recovery goal.
9. Explore and educate about wellness options in community.
10. Educate about peer-support programs in community.
11. Individual expresses his or her health and wellness goal in his or her own words.
12. Individual chooses to move forward on his or her health and wellness goal.

—. _____
_____
—. _____
_____
—. _____
_____

Recovery steps
1. Individual explores his or her hopes and dreams regarding improving and or maintaining health and wellness.
2. Identify how individual sees any mental/co-occurring substance abuse and physical health challenges contributing to the status of his or her health and wellness.
3. Educate individual on various dimensions of health including physical, intellectual, emotional, social, spiritual, environmental, and occupational.
4. Explore with individual specific dimensions of health he or she would like to work on improving and/or maintaining.
5. Individual describes current and/or previous successes and challenges in managing his or her health and wellness.
6. Explore with individual how he or she has historically dealt with the various dimensions of health and wellness.
7. Determine if individual has primary-care physician and has had physical in the past 12 months.

8. Determine if individual has a primary dentist and has had a dental examination in the past 6 months.

9. Individual identifies current challenges to health and wellness (e.g., smoking; drinking too much; over- or undereating; lack of regular physical and dental check-ups and treatment; lack of support; sedentary lifestyle; poor nutrition or finances).

10. Assist individual in identifying and expressing concerns about improving health and wellness.

11. Individual identifies strengths and capacities to support and/or maintain his or her health and wellness.

12. Individual identifies any barriers to improving health and wellness.

13. Determine veteran status.

14. Individual identifies any natural supports her or she wishes to be included in recovery-goal planning meetings.

15. With written permission of the individual, include identified natural supports in recovery-goal planning meetings as individual desires.

16. Identify peer-support organizations available to assist the individual in exploring health and wellness supports.

17. Identify community-based resources to support improving and/or maintain health and wellness.

18. Identify risks and benefits to improving health and wellness.

19. Individual prioritizes one or more dimension of health and wellness to work on.

20. Individual expresses his health and wellness goal in his own words.

21. Individual chooses to move forward with his or her health and wellness goal.

—. _____

_____

—. _____

_____

—. _____

_____

—. _____

_____

—. _____

_____

MOVING FORWARD

Individual's current status

1. Individual has expressed his or her health and wellness goal in his or her own words.
2. Individual has identified and prioritized dimension(s) of health and wellness—including physical, intellectual, emotional, social, spiritual, environmental, occupational—he or she would like to change and or maintain.
3. Primary care physician and date of last physical determined.
4. Primary dentist and date of last dental examination determined.

5. Available history of individual's health and wellness obtained.
6. Individual's current health and wellness activities and strategies identified.
7. Individual's strengths and capacities to improve health and wellness identified.
8. Current barriers to health and wellness identified.
9. Any desired natural supports to be involved in individual's health and wellness recovery goal identified.
10. Individual educated on health and wellness options in community.
11. Individual educated on peer-support programs in community.
12. Individual has chosen to move forward on his or her health and wellness goal.

___. _____

_____

___. _____

_____

Short-term objectives

1. Identify specific plans of action for each of the individual's prioritized wellness dimensions.
2. Link to community resources to support health and wellness recovery goal.
3. Actively engage in utilizing linked resources.
4. Increase use of natural supports.
5. Actively implementing health and wellness recovery goal.

___. _____

_____

_____. _____
       _____
       _____
_____. _____
       _____

Recovery steps

1. Review with individual the specific health and wellness dimensions that they have identified and the priority to work on.
2. Develop together with individual a plan of action for each of his or her priority health and wellness dimensions.
3. Solicit individual's decision about utilizing a peer-support organization and if so, link to same.
4. Obtain signed release of information to make referral to peer-support organization as applicable.
5. Offer enrollment in a Medicaid Health Home, if available.
6. Link to primary care physician to conduct annual physical exam, recommended annual preventative tests and to educate on important health indicators (i.e., cholesterol; blood pressure; BMI; STDs).
7. Link individual to primary dental provider to promote wellness.
8. Assist in helping individual make a list of questions he or she might have for his or her primary care physician and/or dentist.
9. Role-play asking questions from individual's list of questions for primary care physician and/or dentist to prepare individual for medical appointments.
10. Accompany individual to his or her first medical/dental office visit, if desired.
11. Link to Compeer program for social support if desired.
12. Link to stress-management program if desired.
13. Link to community education class on health and wellness topics of interest.
14. Utilize a journal daily to identify positives in one's life.
15. Keep a journal in which you imagine and write about your hopes and dreams for recovery.
16. Identify a possible new friendship and invest time and energy in developing it.
17. Encourage individual to replay in his or her mind days that are happy and enjoy those memories.

18. Link to church, synagogue, mosque, or other as desired by individual.
19. Link to meditation class or group if desired.
20. Link to relaxation class or group if desired.
21. Link to massage therapist or massage therapy school with students in training if desired.
22. Link to mindfulness meditation class or group if desired.
23. Link to yoga class or group if desired.
24. Link to spiritual advisor if desired.
25. Encourage individual to prioritize keeping the company of individuals who do not add stress to his or her lives.
26. Promote the individual taking advantage of available recreational opportunities and the enjoyment that can bring.
27. Discuss and encourage with individual selecting environmentally responsible activities for themselves (i.e., recycling; walking; volunteering time to worthy green causes).
28. Explore with individual strategies for balancing work, family, and personal life.
29. Assist individual in identifying the value of his or her work and/or volunteerism and increasing satisfaction with same.
30. Explore readiness for becoming a peer advocate.
31. Support individual in identifying and engaging in stimulating mental activities (e.g., reading books, newspapers, websites; acquiring a new hobby; learning a new skill; looking for opportunities to be creative).
32. Encourage individual to speak to primary care physician about safe sex practices and birth control/family planning.
33. Where indicated and desired, link to tobacco cessation program.
34. Where indicated and desired, link to a chemical dependency program.
35. With permission, consult with the individual's primary care physician to assist in developing and establishing an exercise routine.
36. Link to a nutritionist for healthy meal planning if desired.
37. Link to primary dental provider to conduct semiannual dental care and to education on important oral health indicators (e.g., gum disease; oral cancer; link between oral health and heart disease).
38. Link to YMCA/YWCA recreational programs and assist in scholarship paperwork where indicated and requested by individual.

39. If veteran, identify and link Veteran's Administration wellness programs.
40. Assist individual in developing strategies to utilize his or her strengths and capacities to overcome any barriers to achieving his or her health and wellness goal.
41. Establish regular meetings with individual to support his or her engagement with established linkages.
42. Encourage ongoing utilization of peer support.
43. Encourage use of natural supports.

—. _____
   _____
—. _____
   _____
—. _____
   _____
—. _____
   _____
—. _____
   _____

LEAVING YOUR PRACTITIONER BEHIND (USING NATURAL ENVIRONMENTS)

Individual's current status
1. Actively implementing health and wellness recovery goal.
2. Linked to community resources to support health and wellness recovery goal, including primary care and dental providers.
3. Individual is utilizing strengths to address any barriers to change.
4. Actively engaged in utilizing linked resources.
5. Beginning to use natural supports.

—. _____
   _____
—. _____
   _____

Short-term objectives
1. Individual maintains engagement and satisfaction with health and wellness opportunities and supports.

2. Individual taking primary responsibility for moving forward on recovery goal utilizing the support of community linkages and natural supports.
3. Individual takes responsibility for his or her health and wellness goal and has knowledge of where to obtain support if they desire to revise his or her goal in the future.

___. _____
_____
___. _____
_____
___. _____
_____

Recovery steps
1. Individual shifts focus from direct work to as-needed problem solving with the practitioner on his or her health and wellness recovery goal.
2. Individual identifies which established community linkages and natural supports he or she wishes to continue independently.
3. Individual consults with practitioner as needed.

___. _____
_____
___. _____
_____
___. _____
_____
___. _____
_____
___. _____
_____

CHAPTER 12   COMMUNITY INVOLVEMENT

A community involvement recovery goal is developed by the individual to assist him or her with expanding his or her life experiences within the community and enriching his or her opportunities for enjoyment and meaning in support of his or her recovery.

INDIVIDUAL'S RECOVERY FOCUS

1. Increased community involvement.

___. _____

_____

___. _____

_____

BEGINNINGS

Individual's current status

1. Lack of community involvement beyond mental health services.
2. Limited community involvement beyond mental health services.
3. Dissatisfied with current level and/or type of community involvement.

___. _____

_____

___. _____

_____

Short-term objectives

1. Individual explores his or her hopes and dreams regarding community involvement.
2. Explore past community involvement experiences.
3. Identify community involvement interests.
4. Individual identifies his or her strengths and capacities to support community involvement.
5. Individual identifies his or her barriers to community involvement.

6. Individual identifies any natural supports (family/significant others and/or friends) he or she wishes to include in his or her community involvement recovery goal.
7. Educate about peer-support programs in community.
8. Individual expresses his or her community involvement goal in his or her own words.
9. Individual chooses to move forward on his or her community involvement goal.

___. _____
_____
___. _____
_____
___. _____
_____

Recovery steps

1. Individual explores his or her hopes and dreams regarding community involvement.
2. Explore with individual how he or she sees community involvement improving his or her quality of life.
3. Individual identifies his or her strengths and capacities that can be utilized to achieve community involvement recovery goal.
4. Assist individual in identifying and expressing any barriers to increasing his or her involvement in the community.
5. Individual lists his or her past community involvement experiences.
6. Individual describes current and/or previous successes and challenges in community environments.
7. Determine veteran status and any current community involvement specific for veterans the individual is participating in.
8. Individual identifies any natural supports he or she wishes to include in his or her community involvement recovery-goal planning meetings.
9. With written permission of the individual, include identified natural supports in recovery-goal planning meetings, as individual desires.
10. Identify the value of working with a peer-support program.
11. Identify risks and benefits to increasing community involvement.
12. Identify range and types of community involvement opportunities.

13. Individual expresses his or her community involvement recovery goal in his or her own words.
14. Individual chooses to move forward on his or her community involvement recovery goal.

—. _____
_____

—. _____
_____
_____

—. _____
_____

—. _____
_____

—. _____
_____

MOVING FORWARD

Individual's current status

1. Individual has expressed his or her community involvement goal in his or her own words.
2. Individual's strengths and capacities to support community involvement identified.
3. Any barriers to community involvement identified.
4. Individual has chosen any natural supports they would like to be involved in his or her community involvement recovery-goal planning meetings.
5. Aware of peer-support programs in community.
6. Individual has chosen to move forward on his or her community involvement goal.

—. _____
_____

—. _____
_____

Short-term objectives

1. Link to community resources to support community involvement recovery goal.
2. Actively engaged in utilizing linked resources.
3. Increased use of natural supports.

4. Actively implementing community involvement recovery goal.

—. _____

   _____

—. _____

   _____

—. _____

   _____

Recovery steps
1. Identify with individual enrichment, recreational, and spiritual opportunities of interest available in community, including volunteer opportunities.
2. Encourage individual to explore online community involvement opportunities of interest to him or her.
3. Identify with individual where there is access to computers they can utilize.
4. Identify opportunities (e.g., newspaper, community bulletin board, online searches) of community events and opportunities.
5. Individual to review community events and opportunities weekly to identify activities of interest (e.g., concerts; library; clubs; continuing education courses; art gallery; museums; free lectures; festivals).
6. Link with local YMCA/YWCA for recreational activities and assist with scholarship paperwork as needed.
7. Link with local clubs of interest (e.g., gardening club; softball team; book club; walking club; bowling team).
8. Link with church, synagogue, mosque, or other organized religious group of interest.
9. Discuss volunteer opportunities in the community.
10. Link to any volunteer opportunity of interest.
11. Link with a local volunteer registry.
12. Encourage individual to personally visit community opportunities of interest and offer to accompany him or her, should he or she choose.
13. Discuss individual's view of the pros and cons of each community opportunity.
14. Assist individual in developing strategies to utilize his or her strengths and capacities to overcome any barriers to achieving his or her community involvement goal.

15. Provide overview of local Compeer Program or other similar programs.
16. Solicit individual's interest about participating in Compeer Program or other similar program and if individual is amenable, obtain a release of information and make referral.
17. Accompany to Compeer Program or other similar program intake interview, if desired.
18. If individual is a veteran, explore veteran-specific community opportunities.
19. Link to any veteran opportunities of interest and accompany if desired.
20. Review peer-support programs options.
21. Solicit individual's decision about utilizing peer support, and if individual is amenable, link to a peer-support agency.
22. Obtain signed release of information to make referral to peer-support agency.
23. Determine individual's decision regarding one or more specific community opportunities to fulfill his or her goal.
24. Support individual in contacting community opportunities of choice and navigating involvement process.
25. Support individual in identifying any required financial costs and problem solve funding needs, as necessary.
26. Support individual in identifying any transportation barriers and problem solve as needed.
27. Establish regular meetings with individual to support his or her engagement with established linkages.
28. Encourage ongoing utilization of peer support.
29. Encourage use of natural supports.

___. _____
    _____
___. _____
    _____
___. _____
    _____
___. _____
    _____
___. _____
    _____

LEAVING YOUR PRACTITIONER BEHIND (USING NATURAL ENVIRONMENTS)

Individual's current status

1. Actively implementing community involvement recovery goal.
2. Linked to community resources to support community involvement recovery goal.
3. Actively engaged in utilizing linked resources.
4. Beginning to use natural supports.

___. _____
_____
___. _____
_____

Short-term objectives

1. Individual maintains engagement and satisfaction with community involvement opportunities and supports.
2. Individual takes primary responsibility for moving forward on community involvement recovery goal, utilizing the support of community linkages and natural supports.
3. Individual takes responsibility for his or her community involvement goal and has knowledge of where to obtain support if he or she desires to revise his or her goal in the future.

___. _____
_____
___. _____
_____
___. _____
_____

Recovery steps

1. Individual shifts focus from direct work to as-needed problem solving with the practitioner on his or her community involvement goal.
2. Individual identifies which established community linkages and natural supports he or she wishes to continue independently.
3. Encourage independent use of peer services to support community involvement recovery goal.

4. Individual consults with practitioner as needed.

___. _____

_____

___. _____

_____

___. _____

_____

___. _____

_____

___. _____

_____

CHAPTER 13   STRESS MANAGEMENT

A stress management recovery goal is developed by the individual to assist him or her with reducing stressors that impact his or her life by enhancing his or her coping skills and community supports in support of the individual's recovery.

INDIVIDUAL'S RECOVERY FOCUS

1. Reduce and cope with stress.

___. _____

   _____

___. _____

   _____

BEGINNINGS

Individual's current status

1. No stress management skills.
2. Minimal stress management skills.
3. Underutilized stress management skills.

___. _____

   _____

___. _____

   _____

Short-term objectives

1. Individual expresses his or her hopes and dreams regarding reducing and coping with stress.
2. Individual identifies current life stressors.
3. Explore how individual has historically dealt with stress.
4. Identify individual's strengths and capacities for healthy stress management.
5. Identify how individual currently copes with stress.
6. Individual identifies current unhealthy ways of dealing with stress.

7. Individual identifies any natural supports (family/significant others and/or friends) he or she would like to be involved in his or her stress management recovery goal.
8. Educate on stress management options in community.
9. Educate on peer-support programs in community.
10. Individual expresses his or her stress management goal in his or her own words.
11. Individual chooses to move forward with his or her stress management goal.

__. _____
_____
__. _____
_____
__. _____
_____

Recovery steps
1. Individual identifies life stressors including how he or she sees any mental, substance abuse, and physical health challenges contributing to his or her current stressors.
2. Inventory with individual how he or she has historically dealt with stress.
3. Individual describes current and/or previous successes and challenges in stress management.
4. Individual identifies strengths and capacities for healthy stress management.
5. Individual identifies any barriers to reducing and coping with stress.
6. Individual identifies current unhealthy ways of dealing with stress (e.g., smoking; drinking too much; over- or undereating; withdrawing from friends, family, and activities; using pills or drugs to relax).
7. Assist individual in identifying and expressing concerns about changing stress management strategies.
8. Determine individual's veteran status and any current veteran's stress management or support programs being utilized.
9. Individual identifies any natural supports he or she wishes to include in his or her recovery-goal planning meetings.

10. With written permission of the individual, include identified natural supports in recovery-goal planning meetings, as individual desires.

11. Identify peer-support organizations available to assist the individual in exploring stress management supports and activities in the community.

12. Identify available community resources to support stress management (e.g., support groups; exercise programs).

13 Identify risks and benefits to changing stress management mechanisms.

14. Individual expresses stress management recovery goal in his or her own words.

15. Individual chooses to move forward on his or her stress management recovery goal.

__. _____
    _____
    _____
__. _____
    _____
    _____
__. _____
    _____
    _____
__. _____
    _____
    _____
__. _____
    _____

MOVING FORWARD

Individual's current status

1. Individual has expressed his or her stress management goal in his or her own words.
2. Individual has identified current life stressors.
3. History of approaches to dealing with stress identified.
4. Current stress management skills identified.
5. Individual strengths and capacities for healthy stress management identified.
6. Current unhealthy ways of dealing with stress identified.
7. Any natural supports the individual would like to be involved in his or her stress management recovery goal identified.
8. Community stress management supports and activities identified.

9. Available peer-support programs identified in community.
10. Individual has chosen to move forward on his or her stress management goal.

___. _____
_____
___. _____
_____

Short-term objectives
1. With individual identify his or her specific stress management plan.
2. Link to community resources to support stress management recovery goal.
3. Actively engaged in utilizing linked resources.
4. Increase use of natural supports.
5. Actively implementing stress management recovery goal.

___. _____
_____
___. _____
_____
___. _____
_____

Recovery steps
1. Explore with individual healthy ways of managing stress (e.g., avoiding unnecessary stress; accepting things the individual cannot change; making time for fun and relaxation; adopting a healthy lifestyle).
2. Discuss individual's view of pros and cons of each identified way of managing stress.
3. Solicit individual's decision about utilizing a peer-support organization and, if so, link to same.
4. Obtain signed release of information to make referral to peer-support organization as applicable.
5. Link individual to a primary care physician or refer to his or her own primary care physician if already linked to assess/address health issues that may be sources of stress.
6. Recommend individual keep a stress journal that identifies regular stressors in his or her life and his or her related coping strategies.

7. Review stress journal regularly together with individual to identify patterns and alternative ways of managing stress.
8. Explore community-based strategies and resources to support stress management (e.g., stress management group; yoga group; mindfulness meditation group; relaxation group; nutrition education).
9. Link to massage therapist or massage therapy school with students in training as available and desired.
10. Link to YMCA/YWCA recreational programs and assist in scholarship paperwork where indicated and requested by individual.
11. Link to smoking cessation group as applicable and desired.
12. Link to substance abuse treatment if coping strategies have included problematic alcohol and/or substance use.
13. Identify healthy ways to relax (e.g., call a friend; go for a walk; take a warm bath; listen to music; play with a pet).
14. If individual is a veteran, identify and link to Veteran's Administration support services.
15. Assist individual in developing strategies to utilize his or her strengths and capacities to overcome any barriers to achieving his or her stress management goal.
16. Establish regular meetings with individual to support his or her engagement with established linkages.
17. Encourage ongoing utilization of peer support.
18. Encourage use of natural supports.

—. _____
    _____
—. _____
    _____
—. _____
    _____
—. _____
    _____
—. _____
    _____

LEAVING YOUR PRACTITIONER BEHIND (USING NATURAL ENVIRONMENTS)

Individual's current status

1. Actively implementing stress management recovery goal.
2. Linked to community resources to support stress management recovery goal.
3. Individual is utilizing strengths to address any barriers to change.
4. Actively engaged in utilizing linked resources.
5. Beginning to use natural supports.

__. _____
   _____
__. _____
   _____

Short-term objectives

1. Individual maintains engagement and satisfaction with stress management opportunities and supports.
2. Individual is taking primary responsibility for moving forward on recovery goal, utilizing the support of community linkages and natural supports.
3. Individual takes responsibility for his or her stress management recovery goal and has knowledge of where to obtain support if he or she desires to revise his or her goal in the future.

__. _____
   _____
__. _____
   _____
__. _____
   _____

Recovery steps

1. Individual shifts focus from direct work to as-needed problem solving with the practitioner on his or her stress management goal.
2. Individual identifies which established community linkages and natural supports he or she wishes to continue independently.

3. Individual consults with practitioner as needed.

—. _____
    _____
—. _____
    _____
—. _____
    _____
—. _____
    _____
—. _____
    _____

CHAPTER 14   RELAPSE PREVENTION

A relapse-prevention recovery goal is developed by the individual to assist him or her with managing his or her overall mental health by minimizing relapses and maximizing his or her recovery.

INDIVIDUAL'S RECOVERY FOCUS

1. Reduce and/or prevent relapse.

___. _____

_____

___. _____

_____

BEGINNINGS

Individual's current status

1. No relapse-prevention plan or skills in place.
2. Minimal relapse-prevention plan or skills in place.
3. Current relapse-prevention plan has not been reviewed and updated within the past 6 months or skills practiced.

___. _____

_____

___. _____

_____

Short-term objectives

1. Individual expresses his or her hopes and dreams regarding reducing and preventing relapse.
2. Individual assesses the effectiveness of his or her current relapse-prevention plan.
3. Explore with individual his or her relapse history.
4. Individual identifies issues/symptoms related to his or her mental/physical health that they associate with relapse.

5. Individual identifies triggers and/or stressors associated with relapse.
6. Individual identifies what has been helpful in past to reduce and/or prevent relapse.
7. Individual identifies what has not been helpful in past to reduce and/or prevent relapse.
8. Identify with individual any natural supports (family/significant others and/or friends) they would like to be involved in his or her relapse-prevention recovery goal.
9. Educate individual on crisis-support services in community.
10. If agreed and needed, add a personal crisis-planning goal to recovery plan (see Chapter 15).
11. With individual, explore peer-support programs in community.
12. Individual has expressed his or her relapse-prevention recovery goal in his or her own words.
13. Individual chooses to move forward on his or her relapse-prevention recovery goal.

___. _____
    _____
___. _____
    _____
___. _____
    _____

Recovery steps

1. Explore with individual his or her hopes and dreams regarding reducing and/or preventing relapse.
2. Individual identifies any current relapse-prevention plan being utilized.
3. Individual identifies where current plan has been successful.
4. Individual identifies where current plan has not been unsuccessful.
5. Review with individual his or her relapse history and patterns that are associated with relapse.
6. Individual identifies issues/symptoms with his or her mental/physical health that he or she associates with relapse.
7. Individual identifies triggers and/or stressors associated with relapse.
8. Individual identifies and lists what has been helpful in past to reduce and/or prevent relapse.

9. Individual identifies and lists what has not been helpful in past to reduce and/or prevent relapse.
10. Provide individual with an overview of all crisis-support services in community and contact information for each.
11. Develop a crisis plan with individual that includes his or her 24/7 crisis-support resource choice.
12. Determine individual's veteran status.
13. Individual identifies any natural supports he or she would like to include in his or her recovery-goal planning meetings.
14. With written permission of the individual, include identified natural supports in recovery planning meetings, as individual desires.
15. Identify peer-support organizations available in the community to assist individual in relapse prevention.
16. Individual expresses his or her relapse-prevention goal in his or her own words.
17. Individual chooses to move forward on his or her relapse-prevention goal.

—. _____
_____
—. _____
_____
—. _____
_____
—. _____
_____
—. _____

MOVING FORWARD

Individual's current status:
1. Individual has expressed his or her relapse-prevention goal in his or her own words.
2. Current relapse-prevention plan assessed.
3. Relapse history gathered and relapse patterns identified.
4. Individual has identified any issues/symptoms with his or her mental/physical health that he or she associates with relapse.
5. Triggers and/or stressors associated with relapse identified.

6. Individual has identified what has been helpful in past to reduce and/or prevent relapse.
7. Individual has identified what has not been helpful in past to reduce and/or prevent relapse.
8. Any natural supports the individual would like to have involved in his or her relapse-prevention recovery goal identified.
9. Individual is aware of crisis-support services in community and specific contact information.
10. Individual's crisis plan developed.
11. Individual is aware of peer-support programs in community.
12. Individual has chosen to move forward on his or her relapse-prevention goal.

___. _____
    _____
___. _____
    _____

Short-term objectives
1. Assist individual in developing his or her relapse plan.
2. With individual, identify skills to support relapse plan and practice same.
3. Link individual to community resources to support relapse-prevention recovery goal.
4. Individual is actively engaged in utilizing linked resources.
5. Individual is increasing use of natural supports.
6. Individual is actively implementing relapse-prevention recovery goal.

___. _____
    _____
___. _____
    _____
___. _____
    _____

Recovery steps
1. Individual identifies any issues/symptoms with his or her mental/physical health that he or she associates with relapse.
2. Individual identifies and list stressors that have put him or her in crisis and relapse.

3. Individual identifies alternative methods to handle stressful events in the future (e.g., avoiding stressful situations; utilizing family and friends for support; engaging in an alternative relaxing activity).

4. Individual identifies current stressors.

5. With individual, develop a stress management recovery goal as indicated (see Chapter 13).

6. Individual identifies strengths and capacities he or she can utilize to support his or her relapse-prevention plan.

7. Identify with individual a list of friends/family members with telephone numbers they can call on a regular basis.

8. Individual identifies a daily community/leisure/healing activity they can engage in to prevent relapse (e.g., walking, meditation, playing cards with a friend).

9. Individual identifies one or more activities associated with past experience of relapse to avoid.

10. Individual identifies specific strategies he or she will take to prevent relapse when there are beginning symptoms/warning signs (e.g., phone a friend; avoid stressful situations; engage in a stress-reducing activity; get ample rest).

11. Individual identifies specific strategies he or she will take if he or she begins to relapse (e.g., review written relapse plan and utilize steps; if applicable, assure medication is being taking on time and in proper dosage; contact his or her mental health counselor; utilize peer supports; contact friends/family).

12. As applicable, individual identifies medication-management self-care techniques (e.g., medications organized by day and time; associate taking medication with a daily activity that triggers a reminder to take medication; develop a method to assure a new prescription refill sufficiently in advance that there is no lapse in available medication).

13. Finalize with individual his or her written relapse prevention plan and provide him or her with a copy.

14. With individual, review and practice as necessary the steps they have identified to prevent relapse and to address when a relapse is occurring.

15. Solicit individual's decision about utilizing a peer-support organization and if individual is amenable, link to same.

16. Obtain signed release of information to make referral to peer-support organization as applicable.
17. If individual is a veteran, identify and link to Veteran's Administration support services.
18. Assist individual in developing strategies to utilize his or her strengths and capacities to support his or her relapse-prevention recovery goal.
19. Establish regular meetings with individual to support his or her engagement with established linkages.
20. Encourage ongoing utilization of peer support.
21. Encourage use of natural supports.

___. _____
   _____
___. _____
   _____
___. _____
   _____
___. _____
   _____
___. _____
   _____

LEAVING YOUR PRACTITIONER BEHIND (USING NATURAL ENVIRONMENTS)

Individual's current status

1. Individual is actively implementing relapse prevention plan.
2. Individual is utilizing his or her strengths and capacities to support implementation of his or her relapse prevention plan.
3. Individual is actively engaged in utilizing linked resources.
4. Individual is engaged and satisfied with current relapse prevention recovery goal.
5. Individual is beginning to use natural supports.

___. _____
   _____
___. _____
   _____

Short-term objectives
1. Individual maintains engagement and satisfaction with relapse-prevention plan.
2. Individual is taking primary responsibility for utilizing supports as outlined in plan.
3. Individual takes ownership of his or her relapse-prevention plan and has knowledge of where to obtain support if he or she desires to revise his or her relapse-prevention recovery goal in the future.
4. Increased use of natural supports.

—. _____

—. _____

—. _____

Recovery steps
1. Individual shifts focus from direct work to as-needed problem solving with the practitioner on issues that arise with his or her relapse-prevention recovery goal.
2. Individual identifies which established community linkages and natural supports he or she wishes to continue independently.
3. Encourage independent use of peer services to support relapse-prevention plan.
4. Individual consults with practitioner as needed.

—. _____

—. _____

—. _____

—. _____

—. _____

CHAPTER 15 PERSONAL CRISIS PLANNING

A personal crisis plan is developed by the individual to define who should take over for him or her and what the individual wants and doesn't want in the way of care and treatment in a crisis. A crisis is a short period of time when an individual may not be able to make decisions in his or her best interest due to a mental health challenge beyond an individual's control.

INDIVIDUAL'S RECOVERY FOCUS

1. To develop a personal crisis plan.

—. _____

   _____

—. _____

   _____

BEGINNINGS

Individual's current status
1. No personal crisis plan in place.
2. Partial personal crisis plan in place.
3. Current personal crisis plan has not been reviewed and updated within the past 6 months.

—. _____

   _____

—. _____

   _____

Short-term objectives
1. Determine if individual has a mental health and, as applicable, substance abuse relapse-prevention plan.
2. Define with individual what a crisis is for him or her.
3. Individual expresses his or her hopes and dreams regarding personal crisis planning.

4. Determine with individual if he or she has a current personal crisis plan and advance directives and when they were last reviewed and updated.
5. Determine with individual if current personal crisis plan is complete.
6. Individual assesses whether current personal crisis plan meets his or her present needs.
7. Individual describes the symptoms and behaviors that would indicate his or her crisis plan needs to be activated by his or her designated supporters.
8. Individual identifies any natural supports (family/significant others and/or friends) he or she would like to be involved in his or her personal crisis plan recovery goal meetings.
9. Explore with individual crisis-support services in community.
10. Explore with individual peer-support/advocate programs in community.
11. Individual expresses his or her personal crisis plan recovery goal in his or her own words.
12. Individual chooses to move forward on his or her personal crisis plan recovery goal.

—. _____
   _____
—. _____
   _____
—. _____
   _____

Recovery steps
1. If agreed and needed, add a relapse-prevention plan goal to recovery plan (see Chapter 14).
2. Explore with individual his or her hopes and dreams regarding a personal crisis plan.
3. Individual defines the symptoms and behaviors that demonstrate he or she is in a mental health and/or substance abuse crisis and, therefore, activates his or her personal crisis plan.
4. Identify and review any existing personal crisis plan.
5. Review any existing advanced directives and if individual does not have any, offer opportunity to assist the individual complete his or her advance directives.

6. Individual answers the following questions about the completeness of his or her plan: (a) Does the plan adequately define his or her mental health and, as applicable, substance abuse symptoms/behaviors that would trigger the plan? (b) Does the plan identify the people of his or her choice to support him or her during a crisis, how to reach them, and the actions they should or should not take on the individual's behalf? (c) Does the plan tell others how the individual wants to be treated and by whom if he or she has a mental health crisis? (d) Does the plan tell others who the individual does not want to treat him or her if he or she has a mental health crisis? (e) Does the plan define which treatments the individual does and does not want to receive? (f) Does the plan identify the individual's current mental health providers, medications, as well as what medications work and what medications do not work, dosages, and current insurance? (g) Does the plan define what has and has not worked for the individual in the past? (h) Does the plan define what needs to be taken care of at home in the individual's absence while he or she is in crisis (e.g., mail; bills; family responsibilities; pet care; home care)? and (i) Does the plan describe the individual's symptoms/behaviors and what he or she is able to do that indicates when his or her crisis plan should be deactivated?

7. Determine with individual whether his or her current plan is comprehensive in addressing all the preceding questions to meet his or her anticipated needs in a crisis.

8. If individual has a comprehensive personal crisis plan and advance directives, determine if reviewed and updated within the past 6 months.

9. Individual identifies if current plan has been used and, if so, where plan has been successful.

10. Provide individual with an overview of all crisis-support services in community and contact information for each.

11. Determine individual's veteran status and any related crisis services that have been utilized.

12. Individual identifies any natural supports he or she would like included in recovery goal crisis planning meetings.

13. With written permission of the individual, include identified natural supports in recovery planning meetings, as individual desires.

14. With individual, identify peer-support/advocacy organizations available in the community to support the individual in personal crisis planning and/or during a crisis.
15. Individual expresses his or her personal crisis plan recovery goal in his or her own words.
16. Individual chooses to move forward with his or her personal crisis plan recovery goal.

___. _____

       _____

___. _____

       _____

___. _____

       _____

___. _____

       _____

___. _____

       _____

MOVING FORWARD

Individual's current status

1. Individual has expressed his/her personal crisis-plan recovery goal in his or her own words.
2. Relapse-prevention plan added as a goal in his or her recovery plan, as needed.
3. Individual has identified what a crisis is for him or her.
4. Any existing previous personal crisis plan or advance directives are identified and when either/both were last reviewed and updated.
5. Individual has defined symptoms and behaviors indicating when his or her crisis plan needs to be activated by his or her designated supporters.
6. Individual has identified any person or persons he or she would like to be involved in the development of his or her personal crisis plan.
7. Individual has contact information for crisis-support services in community.
8. Individual is aware of peer-support programs in community.

9. Individual has chosen to move forward with his or her personal crisis plan recovery goal.

—. _____

_____

—. _____

_____

Short-term objectives

1. Develop and/or update personal crisis plan.
2. Identify and recruit willing person or persons individual wishes to have implement his or her personal crisis plan on his or her behalf.
3. Individual identifies mental health and, as applicable, substance abuse providers to provide treatment in time of crisis.
4. Individual provides and reviews with recruited person or persons with a written copy of his or her personal crisis plan and they understand his or her agreed-upon roles and responsibilities.
5. Individual provides his or her current mental health and housing providers with a written copy of his or her personal crisis plan and reviews same with them.

—. _____

_____

—. _____

_____

—. _____

_____

Recovery steps

1. Assist individual in updating/developing a personal crisis plan.
2. Assist individual in updating/developing advance directives if they have chosen to implement same.
3. Individual defines his or her mental health and, as applicable, substance abuse symptoms/behaviors that would trigger his or her personal crisis plan.
4. Individual identifies person or persons whom he or she has chosen and have agreed to support him or her during a crisis.
5. Obtain release of information for each supporter and mental health practitioner designated for use during time of crisis.
6. Contact information identified for each agreed support person.

7. As desired and available, include a peer advocate among supporters.

8. Tasks have been identified to be assumed by each respective support person.

9. Individual has identified family members and others whom he or she does not wish to have involved in his or her personal crisis plan.

10. Preferred providers and facilities identified to provide treatment services in a crisis.

11. Preferred treatment approaches identified by individual based on prior positive outcomes.

12. Treatment approaches refused by individual in time of crisis have been identified (e.g., ECT; certain medications).

13. Current mental health providers, medications, dosages, pharmacy, and insurance information detailed.

14. Individual lists what approaches and/or intervention have or have not worked for him or her during past crises.

15. What tasks need to be taken care of at the individual's home during a crisis are identified and which supporter has agreed to take responsibility for those tasks in individual's absence (e.g., mail; bills; family responsibilities; pet care; home care).

16. Individual describes what they would be like and what they are able to do that indicates the crisis plan should be deactivated.

17. Finalize with individual his or her written personal crisis plan and provide him or her with copy that has spaces for signatures of each of his or her supporters, his or her primary mental health provider, and current practitioner developing plan with the individual.

18. Individual reviews personal crisis plan when obtaining each desired signature and provides each signatory with a completed copy of his or her plan.

19. Encourage ongoing utilization of peer support and advocacy.

—. _____

_____

—. _____

_____

—. _____

_____

— . _____
_____
— . _____
_____

LEAVING YOUR PRACTITIONER BEHIND (USING NATURAL ENVIRONMENTS)

Individual's current status

1. As agreed, individual has a relapse-prevention plan goal in recovery plan.
2. Individual has a comprehensive crisis plan that has been shared with all agreed supporters and primary mental health provider(s).
3. Every 6 months, individual is initiating a personal crisis plan review and updating as indicated.
4. Individual is linked to available peer-support/advocacy resources to support personal crisis plan.

— . _____
_____
— . _____
_____

Short-term objectives

1. Individual maintains good, ongoing, and frequent communication with identified supports in his or her personal crisis plan.
2. Individual is taking primary responsibility for managing his or her mental and physical health in a manner that reduces the risk of relapse and/or crisis.
3. Individual takes responsibility for his or her personal crisis plan recovery goal and has knowledge of where to obtain support if he or she desires to revise his or her goal in the future.

— . _____
_____
— . _____
_____
— . _____
_____

Recovery steps

1. Individual shifts focus from direct work to as-needed problem solving with the practitioner on issues that arise with his or her crisis plan.
2. Individual identifies which established community linkages and natural supports he or she wishes to continue independently that reduce the risk of relapse and crisis.
3. Individual consults with practitioner as needed.

—. _____
   _____
—. _____
   _____
—. _____
   _____
—. _____
   _____
—. _____
   _____

CHAPTER 16   TRANSPORTATION

A transportation recovery goal is developed by the individual to assist him or her with maximizing his or her access to the community and its resources in support of the individual's recovery.

INDIVIDUAL'S RECOVERY FOCUS

1. Expand community access.

___. _____
      _____
___. _____
      _____

BEGINNINGS

Individual's current status
1. No transportation options.
2. Inadequate transportation options.
3. Underutilized transportation options.

___. _____
      _____
___. _____
      _____

Short-term objectives
1. Individual expresses his or her hopes and dreams regarding transportation.
2. Individual identifies any special accommodations that may be required for transportation.
3. Individual provides transportation history.
4. Individual identifies his or her strengths and capacities to increase transportation possibilities.
5. Individual identifies his or her barriers to transportation.

6. Individual identifies any natural supports (family/significant others and/or friends) he or she might choose to be involved in his or her transportation recovery goal.
7. Individual is aware of transportation options in community.
8. Individual is aware of peer-support programs in community.
9. Individual expresses transportation recovery goal in his or her own words.
10. Individual chooses to move forward with the transportation recovery goal.

___. _____

_____

___. _____

_____

___. _____

_____

Recovery steps

1. Individual explores his or her hopes and dreams regarding transportation.
2. Explore how individual sees transportation improving his or her quality of life.
3. Explore how individual sees any mental and physical health challenges impacting current transportation issues and/or needs.
4. Individual provides a history of current and previous transportation needs and/or issues.
5. Individual identifies his or her strengths and capacities that can be utilized to achieve his or her transportation recovery goal.
6. Assist individual in identifying barriers to transportation needs.
7. Determine with individual if he or she has any documented medical limitations that would impact transportation.
8. Individual describes current and/or previous successes and challenges in transportation needs.
9. Individual identifies any special accommodations necessary for transportation.
10. Identify with individual any natural supports he or she would like included in the development of his or her transportation recovery goal.
11. With written permission, include identified natural supports in recovery-goal planning meetings, as individual desires.

12. Explore with individual peer-support organizations and/or transportation specialists available to assist the consumer in exploring transportation needs and financial support options (e.g., Medicaid transportation; bus tokens for medical appointments; reduced-fare Medicaid bus passes).
13. Individual identifies risks and benefits in utilizing transportation resources.
14. Individual expresses his/her transportation recovery goal in his or her own words.
15. Individual chooses to move forward with his or her transportation recovery goal.

___. _____
      _____
___. _____
      _____
___. _____
      _____
___. _____
      _____
___. _____
      _____

MOVING FORWARD

Individual's current status

1. Individual has expressed his or her transportation recovery goal in his or her own words.
2. Individual has identified any special accommodations necessary for transportation goal.
3. Documented medical limitations that would impact transportation needs are identified.
4. Individual's strengths and capacities to support change in transportation identified.
5. Individual's barriers to utilize transportation resources identified.
6. Individual has determined any natural supports he or she would like to be involved in the individual's transportation recovery goal.
7. Individual is aware of peer-support options in community.
8. Individual has chosen to move forward on his or her transportation recovery goal.

—. _____
    _____
—. _____
    _____

Short-term objectives
1. Individual identifies the specific change desired in transportation needs.
2. Link individual to natural supports and community resources to support transportation recovery goal.
3. Individual actively engaged in utilizing linked resources.
4. Individual actively implementing transportation recovery goal.

—. _____
    _____
—. _____
    _____
—. _____
    _____

Recovery steps
1. Explore with individual the range of transportation options available (i.e., walking; bicycling; bus; subway; cab; Veteran Administration shuttle service; carpooling; car ownership).
2. Individual discusses his or her view of pros and cons of each identified transportation option.
3. Solicit individual's decision about utilizing peer-support and/or transportation specialist, and if the individual is amenable, link to same.
4. Obtain signed release of information to make referral to peer-support agency and/or transportation specialist.
5. If individual chooses not to utilize a peer-support program and/or transportation specialist, explore alternative strategies and resources to support his or her transportation recovery goal.
6. Link individual to his or her choice of alternative community supports.
7. Adapt transportation options to any documented medical limitations.

8. Determine if individual has appropriate footwear and clothing to support his or her identified transportation options.
9. Refer to community clothing closet as needed.
10. Access a map of locality with public transportation lines identified.
11. Access copy of bus schedules.
12. If individual identifies bicycling as an option, determine if assistance in problem solving is available to access needed equipment.
13. Explore with individual the range of public-transportation options available and the cost of each.
14. If indicated and desired by individual, accompany him or her on practice public transportation trips to support learning and reduce anxiety.
15. Connect with Department of Social Services to apply for Medicaid cab authorization and/or reduced fare Medicaid bus tokens and/or public transportation tokens to support transportation to and from medical appointments as available.
16. If individual is a veteran, link to Veteran's Administration transportation services.
17. Brainstorm with individual strategies for carpooling, including family, friends, peers, and community carpooling programs.
18. Determine if individual has a current driver's license.
19. If individual desires to obtain a driver's license, refer to the Department of Motor Vehicles and accompany as desired by individual to assist with the process.
20. Discuss cost of ownership and maintaining a car within the current finances of the individual.
21. If car ownership is desired, develop a plan to obtain same.
22. Assist individual in developing strategies to utilize his or her strengths and capacities to overcome any barriers to achieving his or her transportation recovery goal.
23. Refer to specific veteran transportation supports, as applicable.
24. Establish regular meetings with individual to support his or her engagement with established linkages.
25. Encourage ongoing utilization of peer support.
26. Encourage use of natural supports.

___. _____
     _____
___. _____
     _____
___. _____
     _____
___. _____
     _____

LEAVING YOUR PRACTITIONER BEHIND (USING NATURAL ENVIRONMENTS)

Individual's current status

1. Individual is actively implementing transportation recovery goal.
2. Individual is linked to community resources to support transportation recovery goal.
3. Individual is utilizing strengths to address barriers to change.
4. Individual is actively engaged in utilizing linked resources.
5. Individual is beginning to use natural supports.

___. _____
     _____
___. _____
     _____

Short-term objectives

1. Individual maintains engagement and satisfaction with transportation opportunities and supports.
2. Individual is taking primary responsibility for moving forward on recovery goal utilizing the support of community linkages and natural supports.
3. Individual takes ownership of his or her transportation recovery goal and has knowledge of where to obtain support if he or she desires to revise his or her goal in the future.

___. _____
     _____
___. _____
     _____
___. _____
     _____

Recovery steps

1. Individual shifts focus from direct work to as-needed problem solving with his or her practitioner on his or her transportation recovery goal.
2. Individual identifies which established community linkages and natural supports he or she wishes to continue independently.
3. Encourage independent use of peer services to support transportation recovery goal.
4. Individual consults with practitioner as needed.

—. _____
   _____
   _____
—. _____
   _____
   _____
—. _____
   _____
   _____
—. _____
   _____
   _____
—. _____
   _____

CHAPTER 17   SOCIAL RELATIONSHIPS

A social-relationships recovery goal is developed by the individual to assist him or her with increasing and/or improving his or her social relationships to positively impact his or her quality of life and support the individual's ongoing recovery.

INDIVIDUAL'S RECOVERY FOCUS

1. To increase and/or improve social relationships.

___. _____
   _____
___. _____
   _____

BEGINNINGS

Individual's current status
1. Lack of relationships beyond behavioral health providers.
2. Minimal social relationships beyond behavioral health providers.
3. Dissatisfying social relationships and/or social life.

___. _____
   _____
___. _____
   _____

Short-term objectives
1. Individual expresses hopes and dreams regarding social relationships and/or social life.
2. Individual identifies how satisfied he or she is with current social relationships.
3. Individual identifies his or her strengths and capacities that can be utilized to support social-relationships goal.
4. Individual identifies his or her barriers to social-relationships recovery goal (i.e., afraid in crowds; violence in community; weight).

5. Individual identifies any natural supports (family/significant others and/or friends) he or she wishes to include in recovery planning meetings.
6. Individual expresses his or her social-relationships recovery goal in his or her own words.
7. Individual chooses to move forward on his or her social-relationships recovery goal.

___. _____
   _____
___. _____
   _____
___. _____
   _____

Recovery steps

1. Individual explores his or her hopes and dreams regarding social relationships.
2. Individual discusses current social relationships.
3. Individual identifies his or her level of satisfaction with each of his or her current social relationships.
4. Individual explores how his or her mental health challenges have impacted his or her social relationships.
5. With individual, discuss how he or she feels his or her social relationships or the lack thereof, may promote or hinder recovery.
6. Individual explores the challenges and benefits around his or her current social relationships.
7. Individual explores the challenges and benefits to expanding the number of social relationships.
8. Individual expresses how social relationships may or may not improve his or her quality of life.
9. Individual identifies barriers to achieving desired social relationships goal.
10. Identify with individual any natural supports he or she would like included in development of his or her social-relationships recovery goal.
11. With written permission, include identified natural supports in recovery-goal planning meetings, as individual desires.
12. Individual expresses his or her social-relationships recovery goal in his or her own words.

13. Individual chooses to move forward with his or her social-relationships recovery goal.

___. _____

___. _____

___. _____

___. _____

___. _____

MOVING FORWARD

Individual's current status

1. Individual has expressed his or her social-relationships goal in his or her own words.
2. Individual has identified his or her strengths and capacities to support social-relationships recovery goal.
3. Individual has identified barriers to social-relationships recovery goal.
4. Individual has identified any natural supports he or she wishes to include in recovery planning meetings.
5. Individual has chosen to move forward on his or her social-relationship recovery goal.

___. _____

___. _____

Short-term objectives

1. With individual, identify his or her social-skills strengths and challenges.
2. Explore with individual the full range of informal and formal social-skills-building opportunities and supports available in the community.
3. Link individual to his or her preferred informal and formal social-skills-building opportunities and supports in the community.

___. _____
       _____
___. _____
       _____
___. _____
       _____

Recovery steps

1. Identify with individual the range of informal social skills building opportunities and supports in the community (e.g., community education programs; faith-based programs; self-help groups; Toastmasters Club; YouTube social-skills training videos).

2. Identify with individual the range of peer-support social-skills-building opportunities and supports in the community (e.g., peer counseling/mentoring/coaching; peer-run social-skills training classes; peer-sponsored social events; peer-run support group).

3. Individual identifies any informal social-skills-building opportunities and supports he or she desires to utilize.

4. Assist individual with linkage to his or her preferred informal social-skills-building opportunities and supports, and accompany him or her to initial linkage, if desired.

5. Where individual has requested assistance, obtain signed release of information by the individual to speak with any informal supports.

6. Identify with individual the range of formal social-skills-building opportunities and supports available in community (e.g., individual therapist—private practice or community mental health; social-skills-building group; psycho-education groups; psychiatric rehabilitation program; PROS—Personalized Recovery-Oriented Services; Continuing Day Treatment; Intensive Psychiatric Rehabilitation Treatment).

7. If individual is a veteran, link consumer to Veteran Administration for social-skills-building opportunities and supports, as available and desired.

8. Individual identifies any formal social-skills opportunities and supports they desire to utilize.

9. Obtain signed release of information to facilitate linkage to formal social-skills opportunities and supports.

10. Assist individual with linkage to his or her preferred formal social-skills-building opportunities and supports and accompany him or her to initial linkage if desired.

11. Identify with individual the range of natural, informal, and formal social opportunities to expand potential social relationships that are available in the community that are consistent with his or her interests (e.g., friends/family/peers; clubs focused on special interest; faith-based social activities; community recreation opportunities; volunteer opportunities; community events; online dating services; singles organizations; couples' social events; joint activities with family and/or friends).

12. Assist individual with linkage to his or her preferred social opportunities and accompany him or her to initial linkage if requested.

13. Support individual in identifying any required financial costs for linkages and problem solve funding needs, as necessary.

14. Support individual in identifying any transportation barriers and problem solve as needed.

15. Assist individual in developing strategies to utilize his or her strengths and capacities to overcome any barriers to achieving his or her social relationships recovery goal.

16. Establish regular meetings with individual to support his or her engagement with established linkages.

17. Encourage ongoing use of peer support.

—. _____

—. _____

—. _____

—. _____

—. _____

LEAVING YOUR PRACTITIONER BEHIND (USING NATURAL ENVIRONMENTS)

Individual's current status
1. Individual is linked to desired informal supports.
2. Individual is linked to desired formal supports.
3. Individual is beginning to use natural supports.

4. Individual is engaged and satisfied with current social-relationships recovery goal.

___. _____

   _____

___. _____

   _____

Short-term objectives

1. Individual maintains engagement and satisfaction with social-skills-building opportunities and supports.
2. Individual taking primary responsibility for utilizing natural, informal, and formal social opportunities and skill-building supports.
3. Individual takes responsibility for his or her social relationships recovery goal and has knowledge of where to obtain support if they desire to revise his or her goal in the future.

___. _____

   _____

___. _____

   _____

Recovery steps

1. Individual shifts focus from direct work to as-needed problem solving with his or her practitioner on his or her social-relationships recovery goal.
2. Individual identifies which established informal, formal, and natural supports they wish to continue independently to support his or her social-relationships recovery goal.
3. Individual consults with practitioner as needed.

___. _____

   _____

___. _____

   _____

___. _____

   _____

___. _____

   _____

CHAPTER 18   MEANINGFUL ACTIVITIES

A meaningful-activities recovery goal is developed by the individual to assist him or her with enriching his or her life through a range of activities that provide opportunities for enjoyment as well as making a contribution in the community in support of the individual's recovery.

INDIVIDUAL'S RECOVERY FOCUS

1. Increase involvement in meaningful activities.

—. _____

_____

—. _____

_____

BEGINNINGS

Individual's current status
1. Lack of meaningful activities beyond paid mental health services.
2. Limited meaningful activities beyond paid mental health services.
3. Dissatisfied with current level and/or type of meaningful activities.

—. _____

_____

—. _____

_____

Short-term objectives
1. Individual expresses his or her hopes and dreams regarding meaningful activities.
2. Individual identifies meaningful activities of interest to him or her.
3. Individual identifies his or her strengths and capacities to support meaningful activities.
4. Individual identifies any barriers to participating in meaningful activities.

5. Individual identifies any natural supports (family/significant others and/or friends) he or she might choose to be involved in his or her meaningful-activities recovery goal.
6. Educate about peer-support programs in community.
7. Individual expresses his or her meaningful-activities recovery goal in his or her own words.
8. Individual chooses to move forward on his or her meaningful-activities recovery goal.

___. _____
   _____
___. _____
   _____
___. _____
   _____

Recovery steps

1. Explore with individual his or her hopes and dreams regarding meaningful activities.
2. Explore how individual sees meaningful activities improving his or her quality of life.
3. Individual identifies his or her strengths and capacities that can be utilized to achieve meaningful-activities recovery goal.
4. Assist individual in identifying any barriers to increasing his or her participation in meaningful activities.
5. List past meaningful activities that have been most satisfying to individual.
6. Individual describes current and/or previous successes and challenges to engaging in meaningful activities.
7. Determine individual's veteran status and any current or previous veteran activities involvement.
8. Individual identifies any natural supports they choose to be involved in his or her meaningful-activities recovery goal.
9. With written permission, include identified natural supports in recovery-goal planning meetings, as individual desires.
10. Identify the value of working with a peer-support program.
11. Identify risks and benefits to increasing meaningful activities.
12. Identify kinds and scope of meaningful-activity opportunities.
13. Individual expresses his or her meaningful activities recovery goal in his or her own words.

14. Individual chooses to move forward with his or her meaningful-activities recovery goal.

__. _____
   _____

__. _____
   _____

__. _____
   _____

__. _____
   _____

__. _____
   _____

MOVING FORWARD

Individual's current status
1. Individual has expressed his or her meaningful-activities goal in his or her own words.
2. Meaningful activities of interest explored.
3. Individual's strengths and capacities to support meaningful activities identified.
4. Individual has identified any barriers to participating in meaningful activities.
5. Individual has chosen any natural supports he or she would like to be involved in his or her meaningful-activities recovery goal.
6. Individual is aware of peer-support programs in community.
7. Individual has chosen to move forward on his or her meaningful-activities goal.

__. _____
   _____

__. _____
   _____

Short-term objectives
1. Identify specific meaningful activities to support goal.
2. Link to community resources to support meaningful-activities recovery goal.
3. Actively engaged in utilizing linked resources.
4. Increase use of natural supports.

5. Actively implementing meaningful-activities recovery goal.

—. _____
   _____
—. _____
   _____
—. _____
   _____

Recovery steps

1. Brainstorm with individual the range of potential meaningful activities.
2. Educate individual about how meaningful activities can be in the home as well as in the community (e.g., reading, cleaning your home, yard work; inviting a friend to play cards).
3. Encourage individual to explore online meaningful activities of interest to him or her.
4. Assist individual in identifying where there is computer access in the community he or she can utilize.
5. Identify opportunities (e.g., newspaper, community bulletin board, online searches) of meaningful activities in the community.
6. Individual identifies up to three meaningful activities he or she would like to engage in.
7. Individual discusses the opportunities and challenges associated with each meaningful activity of choice.
8. Encourage individual to personally visit community opportunities of interest and offer to accompany him or her should they desire.
9. Assist individual in developing strategies to utilize his or her strengths and capacities to overcome any barriers to achieving his or her meaningful activities recovery goal.
10. If individual is a veteran, explore veteran-specific meaningful-activity opportunities.
11. Link to any veteran opportunities of interest and accompany if desired.
12. Review peer-support program options.
13. Solicit individual's decision about utilizing peer support, and if individual is amenable, link to a peer-support agency.
14. Obtain signed release of information to make referral to peer-support agency if desired.

15. Support individual in contacting meaningful activities of choice and navigating involvement process.
16. Support individual in identifying any required financial costs and problem solve funding needs as necessary.
17. Support individual in identifying any transportation barriers and problem solve as needed.
18. Establish regular meetings with individual to support his or her engagement with established linkages.
19. Encourage ongoing utilization of peer support.
20. Encourage use of natural supports.

—. _____
_____
—. _____
_____
—. _____
_____
—. _____
_____
—. _____
_____

LEAVING YOUR PRACTITIONER BEHIND (USING NATURAL ENVIRONMENTS)

Individual's current status
1. Individual is actively implementing his or her meaningful-activities recovery goal.
2. Individual is linked to community resources to support meaningful-activities goal.
3. Actively engaged in utilizing linked resources.
4. Individual is utilizing his or her strengths and capacities to address any barriers to change.
5. Beginning to use natural supports in community.

—. _____
_____
—. _____
_____
—. _____
_____

Short-term objectives

1. Individual continues engagement and satisfaction with meaningful activities and supports he or she is utilizing.
2. Individual is taking primary responsibility for moving forward on his or her meaningful-activities recovery goal utilizing community linkages and natural supports.
3. Individual takes responsibility for his or her meaningful-activities recovery goal and has knowledge of where to obtain support if he or she desires to revise his or her goal in the future.

___. _____
_____
___. _____
_____
___. _____
_____

Recovery steps

1. Individual shifts focus from direct work to as-needed problem solving with the practitioner on his or her meaningful-activities recovery goal.
2. Individual identifies which established community linkages and natural supports they wish to continue independently.
3. Encourage independent use of peer services to support meaningful-activities recovery goal.
4. Individual consults with practitioner as needed.

___. _____
_____
___. _____
_____
___. _____
_____
___. _____
_____
___. _____
_____

CHAPTER 19   LIFE SKILLS

A life skills recovery goal is developed by the individual to assist him or her with identifying and improving selected life skills (e.g., cooking; personal hygiene; shopping) in pursuit of greater independence and/or safety in support of his or her recovery.

INDIVIDUAL'S RECOVERY FOCUS

1. Increase desired life skills to promote appropriate independence and/or safety.

—. _____

_____

—. _____

_____

BEGINNINGS

Individual's current status

1. Interest in increasing life skills in one or more areas impacting independence and/or safety.

—. _____

_____

—. _____

_____

Short-term objectives

1. Individual expresses hopes and dreams regarding life skills for independence.
2. Individual provides history of prior level of life skills knowledge.
3. Individual's strengths and capacities to support increased life skills are identified.
4. Individual's barriers to increasing life skills are identified.

5. Individual identifies any natural supports (family/significant others and/or friends) they might choose to be involved in his or her life skills recovery goal.
6. Individual aware of peer-support programs in community.
7. Individual has expressed his or her life skills recovery goal in his or her own words.
8. Individual chooses to move forward on his or her life skills recovery goal.

___. _____

   _____

___. _____

   _____

   _____

___. _____

   _____

Recovery steps

1. Explore individual's hopes and dreams regarding increasing life skills.
2. Explore how individual sees increasing life skills improving his or her quality of life.
3. Individual discusses what they would like to know/gain in life skills.
4. Individual identifies his or her strengths and capacities that can be utilized to achieve life skills recovery goal.
5. Assist individual in identifying barriers to increasing his or her life skills.
6. Individual describes current and/or previous successes and challenges in life skills.
7. Determine individual's veteran status for possible veteran linkages.
8. Identify with individual any natural supports he or she would like included in development of his or her life skills recovery goal.
9. With written permission, include identified natural supports in recovery planning meetings, as individual desires.
10. Explore with the individual the value of working with a peer-support program.
11. Individual identifies risks and benefits to increasing life skills.
12. Individual expresses his or her life skills recovery goal in his or her own words.

13. Individual chooses to move forward on his or her life skills recovery goal.

__. _____
   _____
__. _____
   _____
__. _____
   _____
__. _____
   _____
__. _____
   _____

MOVING FORWARD

Individual's current status
1. Individual has expressed his or her life skills recovery goal in his or her own words.
2. Individual has provided history of prior level of life skills knowledge.
3. Individual's strengths and capacities to support increased life skills are identified.
4. Individual's identifies barriers to increasing life skills.
5. Individual has identified any natural supports he or she would like to be involved in his or her life skills recovery goal.
6. Individual is aware of peer-support programs in community.
7. Individual has chosen to move forward on his or her life skills recovery goal.

__. _____
   _____
__. _____
   _____

Short-term objectives
1. Individual identifies his or her priority life skills areas they would like to improve.
2. Individual is aware of informal community supports to improve life skills functioning.

3. Individual is aware of formal community supports to improve life skills functioning.
4. Link to individual's choices of natural, informal, and/or formal community resources to support life skills recovery goal.
5. Individual is actively engaged in utilizing linked resources.
6. Individual is actively implementing life skills recovery goal.

—. _____
   _____
—. _____
   _____
—. _____
   _____

Recovery steps

1. Individual identifies life skills areas for improvement that are his or her recovery-goal priority.
2. Discuss and inform individual on the range of informal life skills supports (e.g., peer support; self-help groups; Club House Model of Psychosocial Rehabilitation; cooking clubs; YouTube life skills educational/demonstration videos [e.g., cooking, laundry, cleaning, grooming, care of pets]; community continuing-education programs).
3. Discuss with and educate individual on the range of peer-support services available in his or her community to increase life skills (e.g., peer mentoring/coaching; peer-run mutual aid groups; peer-run relapse prevention group; peer-run conflict-resolution and skill-building groups; peer-run advocacy group; peer telephone support; peer-run recovery support drop-in centers; peer-run money-management group; peer-run life skills group; peer-run community mobility training; peer-run medication-management group; peer-run safety group; peer-run personal hygiene group; peer-run technology-use group).
4. Discuss with and educate individual on the range of self-help groups available in community to increase life skills (e.g., peer-run groups; veteran self-help group; online life-skills chat group; money-management group; self-defense group; medication-management group; time-management group; nutrition group; health-management and maintenance group; managing-a-household group; coupon-clipping group; parenting group).

5. Individual identifies any informal life skills supports they desire to utilize.
6. Assist individual with linkage to his or her preferred informal life skills supports and accompany him or her to initial linkage if desired.
7. Where individual has requested assistance, obtain signed release of information to speak with any informal supports.
8. Discuss with and inform individual on range of formal life skills supports available in community (e.g., individual therapist—private practice or community mental health—skills-building groups; psycho-education groups; medication management; psychiatric rehabilitation program; PROS—Personalized Recovery Oriented Services; Continuing Day Treatment; habilitation services; Cooperative Extension food, nutrition, and health programs).
9. If individual is a veteran, link individual to Veteran Administration education and self-help programs, as desired.
10. Individual identifies any formal life skills community supports they desire to utilize.
11. Obtain signed release of information from the individual for each preferred formal life skills community support(s) linkage to be made.
12. Link individual to his or her preferred formal life skills community support(s) and accompany him or her to initial linkage, if requested.
13. Assist individual in developing strategies to utilize his or her strengths and capacities to overcome any barriers to achieving his or her life skills recovery goal.
14. Support individual in identifying any required financial costs and problem solve funding needs, as necessary.
15. Support individual in identifying any transportation barriers and problem solve as needed.
16. If desired, assist individual in discussing with identified natural supports how they can assist individual in achieving his or her life skills support goal.
17. Establish regular meetings with individual to support his or her engagement with established linkages.
18. Encourage ongoing utilization of peer support.

—. _____
_____
—. _____
_____
—. _____
_____
—. _____
_____

LEAVING YOUR PRACTITIONER BEHIND (USING NATURAL ENVIRONMENTS)

Individual's current status
1. Individual is linked to desired informal supports.
2. Individual is linked to desired formal supports.
3. Beginning to use natural supports.
4. Actively implementing life skills recovery goal.
5. Individual is engaged and satisfied with current life skills supports.

—. _____
_____
—. _____
_____

Short-term objectives
1. Individual maintains engagement and satisfaction with life skills supports.
2. Individual is taking primary responsibility for utilizing natural, informal, and formal life skills supports.
3. Individual takes ownership of his or her life skills recovery goal and has knowledge of where to obtain support if he or she desires to revise his or her goal in the future.

—. _____
_____
—. _____
_____
—. _____
_____

Recovery steps

1. Individual identifies which established natural, informal, and formal supports he or she wishes to continue independently to support his or her life skills recovery goal.
2. Individual shifts focus from direct work to as-needed problem solving with the practitioner on issues that arise with his or her life skills recovery goal.
3. Individual consults with practitioner as needed.

___. _____
    _____
    _____
___. _____
    _____
    _____
___. _____
    _____
    _____
___. _____
    _____
    _____
___. _____
    _____

APPENDIX: BLANK INDIVIDUAL SERVICE PLAN FORMS

Participant Name: _____
ID: _____ DOB: _____

Care Coordination Program: _____
Date of Plan: _____

INDIVIDUAL SERVICE PLAN

You and your Care Coordinator have the opportunity to work together on an Individual Service Plan (ISP) and a Crisis Prevention Plan. You may also want a friend, a family member, and/or a valued provider included in the development of this plan.

Services in the plan may include mental health and/or chemical dependency treatment, housing and financial assistance, and any other things that you identify as a support. You can also address life areas that you are not satisfied with or need more help with. You may want to set goals and develop a service plan that addresses some or all of the following life areas:

Recovery & Rehabilitation

Physical Health & Wellness

Financial

Housing

Community Presence & Participation

Self-Help & Empowerment

Educational & Employment

Legal

Spirituality

Other _____

You may write a plan with as many goals and services as you want. You may review the plan and add goals and services at any time by talking about this with your Care Coordinator.

Reproduced by Permission of the New York Care Coordination Project, Inc.

Participant Name: _____   Care Coordination Program: _____
ID: _____   DOB: _____   Date of Plan: _____

As you work with your Care Coordinator on the Individual Service Plan, you will want to consider what personal supports and community resources can help you achieve your goals, what services and which service providers have been most helpful in the past, what prevents you from getting and keeping what you need, and what strengths, supports, and experiences you can use to achieve your goals. Your Care Coordinator will assist you in accessing the services, supports, and organizations that you need in order to carry out your plan.

Your Care Coordinator will also work with you to develop a Crisis Prevention Plan. This plan will help you recognize situations and people that may cause you stress, and identify people and things that may help you to relieve stress.

Participant Name: _____

ID: _____   DOB: _____

Part A—Participant's Personal Profile
(As established in the Assessment)

Values and areas of interest (Things that are important to me: hopes, dreams, interests)

Strengths (Skills, qualities, and experiences that can help me achieve my goals)

Participant Name: _____ DOB: _____

Care Coordination Program: _____

ID: _____

Date of Plan: _____

Personal and community supports (People and/or things I have in my life that can help me achieve my goals)

Possible barriers (Things that could prevent me from achieving these goals)

Part A—Participant's Personal Profile (continued)
(As established in the Assessment)

Discharge criteria (How I will know that I don't need Care Coordination anymore)

Participant Name: _____ DOB: _____ Care Coordination Program: _____

ID: _____ Date of Plan: _____

Date	Update Information	Participant Initials	Provider Initials

Participant Name: _____
ID: _____

Care Coordination Program: _____
DOB: _____ Date of Plan: _____

Part A—Participant's Personal Profile (continued)
(As established in the Assessment)

Date	Update Information	Participant Initials	Provider Initials

Copy this page as often as needed to provide updates to the participant's personal profile.

Participant Name: _____

ID: _____ DOB: _____

Care Coordination Program: _____

Date of Plan: _____

Part B—Participant's Goal, Objective, and Services

Goal # _____ Participant's Desired Outcome: _____

Development Date: _____

Barriers (What is getting in the way of achieving the goal as per Assessment)

Strengths (Existing supports for achieving the goal)

Objective # _____ (Step toward the goal and how I will know I have accomplished this)

Effective Date: _____   Target Completion Date: _____

Specific Services/Activities/Supports/Tasks (What I and/or others will do to achieve this objective)	Who is Responsible (Person/s who will provide the service or carry out the task)	Start Date	Target Completion Date	Frequency (How often)	Service $ Expense (CK if yes)

Ongoing Updates

Date	Progress	Achievement Code	Participant Initials	Provider Initials

Copy this page as often as needed to create new goals and/or objectives. Attach additional pages (see next page) as needed to provide updates to this goal and/or objective.

Reproduced by Permission of the New York Care Coordination Project, Inc.

Participant Name: _____   Care Coordination Program: _____

ID: _____   DOB: _____   Date of Plan: _____

Part B—Participant's Goal, Objective, and Services (continued)

Goal # _____   **Participant's Desired Outcome:** _____

Development Date: _____

Objective # _____   (Step toward the goal and how I will know I have accomplished this)

_____

Effective Date: _____   **Target Completion Date:** _____

Ongoing Updates				
Date	**Progress**	**Achievement Code**	**Participant Initials**	**Provider Initials**

Copy this page as often as needed to provide updates to this goal and/or objective.

Participant Name: _____

ID: _____ DOB: _____

Care Coordination Program: _____

Date of Plan: _____

PART C—PARTICIPANT'S CRISIS PREVENTION PLAN

If the participant has a Wellness Recovery Action Plan™ (WRAP), it may be attached and this form used only for additional or updated information.

HEALTH CARE PROXY HAS BEEN EXECUTED? ( ) Yes ( ) No ☐ Copy Attached	OTHER ADVANCE DIRECTIVE HAS BEEN EXECUTED? ( ) Yes ( ) No ☐ Copy Attached	WELLNESS RECOVERY ACTION PLAN™ (WRAP) HAS BEEN EXECUTED? ( ) Yes ( ) No ☐ Copy Attached
Document Location:	Document Location:	Document Location:
Does the Participant have a copy? ( ) Yes ( ) No	Does the Participant have a copy? ( ) Yes ( ) No	Does the Participant have a copy? ( ) Yes ( ) No
If No: ___ Need More Information ___ Refused (state reason below)	If No: ___ Need More Information ___ Refused (state reason below)	If No: ___ Need More Information ___ Refused (state reason below)

MY CRISIS PREVENTION PLAN: (How can I avoid a crisis?):

Are there people, places, or things I should avoid? What are they?

What are my early warning signs?

My CRISIS PLAN (What can be done if I am in crisis?)

Ways I can relieve stress, regain balance, calm myself, or make myself safer:

Persons I can call:	Resources I can use:

Things I or others can do that I find helpful or keep me safe:

Medications that have helped in the past:	Medications that have Not helped:	Types of medication(s) I take:

Participant Name: _____ DOB: _____

Care Coordination Program: _____

ID: _____

Date of Plan: _____

PART C—PARTICIPANT'S CRISIS PREVENTION PLAN (CONTINUED)

IF I BECOME UNABLE TO HANDLE MY PERSONAL AFFAIRS, the following people have agreed to look after my personal affairs (For example: pets, housing, family/job notification):

Name	Phone	Area(s) of Assistance

I have developed this Crisis Plan to describe the actions that I would like to take place should I be in a crisis situation.

Participant's Signature: _____ Date: _____

Ongoing Updates

Review Date	Update / Comment	Participant Initials	Provider Initials

Attach additional pages (see next page) as needed to provide updates to the Crisis Prevention Plan.

Reproduced by Permission of the New York Care Coordination Project, Inc.

Participant Name: _____ Care Coordination Program: _____

ID: _____ DOB: _____ Date of Plan: _____

PART C—PARTICIPANT'S CRISIS PREVENTION PLAN (CONTINUED)

Ongoing Updates

Review Date	Update / Comment	Participant Initials	Provider Initials

Copy this page as often as needed to provide updates to the Crisis Prevention Plan.

Participant Name: _____

ID: _____

Care Coordination Program: _____

DOB: _____

Date of Plan: _____

ASSESSMENT / PLAN SUMMARY / REVIEW—SIGNATURE PAGE

TYPE: Initial Plan: _____ Periodic Review 3 mo _____ Periodic Review 6 mo _____ Other Review _____ Date: _____

Participant Comments (Comment on progress toward goals and topics that require further discussion and/or services that might be further explored.)

Provider Comments (Provide a brief summary of the plan, including identified areas of concern that are not in the ISP, reasons for not including them at this time, and what, if any future actions will be taken to include them. Use this summary to update the assessment, as required.)

Signatures of Individuals Contributing to the Individual Service Plan:

Copies of Plan Provided To:

Participant Signature:	Participant Name:
Date:	Date:
Care Coordinator Signature:	Care Coordinator Name:
Date:	Date:
Service Provider Signature:	Service Provider Name:
Date:	Date:
Other Signature (specify):	Other Name (specify):
Date:	Date:

ABOUT THE AUTHORS

Catherine N. Dulmus, PhD, LCSW, is Professor, Associate Dean for Research, and Director of the Buffalo Center for Social Research at the University at Buffalo, and Research Director at Hillside Family of Agencies in Rochester, New York. She received her baccalaureate degree in social work from Buffalo State College and her master's degree in social work and a doctoral degree in social welfare from the University at Buffalo. As a researcher with interests that include mental health, evidence-based practice, and university-community research partnerships, Dr. Dulmus's recent contributions have focused on fostering interdependent collaborations among practitioners, researchers, schools, and agencies critical in the advancement and dissemination of new and meaningful knowledge. She has published 22 books and over 50 peer-reviewed journal articles. Prior to obtaining the PhD, her social work practice background encompassed almost a decade of experience in the fields of mental health and school social work.

Bruce C. Nisbet, LMSW, is President and CEO of Spectrum Human Services in Orchard Park, New York, a large not-for-profit community mental health agency serving Buffalo, New York, and surrounding counties. In addition, he is President of Health Home Partners of WNY, LLC, a not-for-profit corporate collaboration of three major health-care providers who are designated a Health Home in New York State. Nisbet is also currently a Research Associate with the Buffalo Center for Social Research. His previously held positions include President/CEO of the Children's Home of Wyoming Conference in Binghamton, New York, and Executive Vice President and Chief Program Officer at Gateway-Longview, Inc. in Williamsville, New York, both large comprehensive child welfare agencies. Nisbet holds a baccalaureate degree in philosophy and a master's degree in social work from the University at Buffalo. He is a board member of the New York Council for Community Behavioral Health Care, founder and Past President of the New York State Coalition of 853 Schools and he has been a member of the National Public Policy Committee of the Alliance for Children and Families. He sits on the editorial boards of *Best Practices in Mental Health* and the *Journal of Evidence-Based Social Work,* and his scholarly interests include evidence-based mental health practice, neuroscience, mental health recovery, and university/community partnerships.

ABOUT THE CD-ROM

INTRODUCTION

This appendix provides you with information on the contents of the CD that accompanies this book. For the latest information, please refer to the ReadMe file located at the root of the CD.

SYSTEM REQUIREMENTS

Make sure that your computer meets the minimum system requirements listed in this section. If your computer doesn't match up to most of these requirements, you may have a problem using the contents of the CD.

- A computer with a processor running at 120 Mhz or faster.
- At least 32 MB of total RAM installed on your computer; for best performance, we recommend at least 64 MB.
- A CD-ROM drive.
- Adobe Flash Player 9 or later (free download from Adobe.com).

Note: Many popular word-processing programs are capable of reading Microsoft Word files. However, users should be aware that a slight amount of formatting might be lost when using a program other than Microsoft Word.

USING THE CD WITH WINDOWS

To access the content from the CD, follow these steps:

1. Insert the CD into your computer's CD-ROM drive. The license agreement appears (Windows 7 > Select **Start.exe** from the AutoPlay window or follow the same steps for Windows Vista).
   The interface won't launch if you have autorun disabled. In that case, click Start > Run (for Windows Vista, Start > All Programs > Accessories > Run). In the dialog box that appears, type **D:\Start.exe**. (Replace **D** with the proper letter if your CD drive

uses a different letter. If you don't know the letter, see how your CD drive is listed under My Computer.) Click **OK**.

2. Read through the license agreement, and then click the Accept button if you want to use the CD. The CD interface appears. Simply select the material you want to view.

USING THE CD WITH A MAC

To install the items from your CD to your hard drive, follow these steps:

1. Insert the CD into your computer's CD-ROM drive.
2. The CD icon will display on your desktop; double-click to open it.
3. Double-click the **Start** button.
4. Read the license agreement, and then click the **Accept** button to use the CD.
5. The CD interface will display. The interface provides a simple point-and-click way to explore the contents of the CD.

Note for Mac users: The content menus may not function as expected in newer versions of Safari and Firefox; however, the documents are available by navigating to the Author Files folder.

WHAT'S ON THE CD

The following sections provide a summary of the software and other materials you'll find on the CD.

CONTENT

Includes all recovery goal forms from the book in Word (.doc) format and blank forms from the appendix in Word (.doc) format, reproduced by permission of the New York Care Coordination Project, Inc. These recovery goals and forms can be customized and printed out.

APPLICATIONS

Microsoft Word Viewer

Included on this CD is a link to download Microsoft Word Viewer. Microsoft Word Viewer is a freeware viewer that allows you to view, but not edit, most Microsoft Word files. Certain features of Microsoft Word documents may not display as expected from within Word Viewer.

Troubleshooting

If you have difficulty installing or using any of the materials on the companion CD, try the following solutions:

- Turn off any antivirus software that you may have running. Installers sometimes mimic virus activity and can make your computer incorrectly believe that it is being infected by a virus. (Be sure to turn the antivirus software back on later.)
- Close all running programs. The more programs you're running, the less memory is available to other programs. Installers also typically update files and programs; if you keep other programs running, installation may not work properly.
- Reboot if necessary. If all else fails, rebooting your machine can often clear any conflicts in the system.

Customer Care

If you have trouble with the CD-ROM, please call the Wiley Product Technical Support phone number at (800) 762-2974. Outside the United States, call (317) 572-3994. You can also contact Wiley Product Technical Support at **http://support.wiley.com**. John Wiley & Sons will provide technical support only for installation and other general quality control items. For technical support of the applications themselves, consult the program's vendor or author.

To place additional orders or to request information about other Wiley products, please call (877) 762-2974.